T

AIDS

ACQUIRED IMMUNODEFICIENCY SYNDROME

HANDBOOK

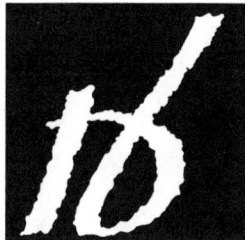

Designbase Publishing
P.O. Box 3601
Durham,
North Carolina
27702-3601

A Division of Designbase Associates, Incorporated

T H E

AIDS

ACQUIRED IMMUNODEFICIENCY SYNDROME

HANDBOOK

A COMPLETE GUIDE TO
Education
and
Awareness

By Brenda S. Faison, M.P.D.
Edited by Laila Moustafa, Ph.D.

Copyright © 1991 by Brenda Smith Faison

All rights reserved. No part of this book may be reproduced or transmitted in any form or by any means, electronic or mechanical, including photocopying, recording or by any informational storage or retrieval system— except by a reviewer who may quote brief passages in a review to be printed in a magazine or newspaper —without permission in writing from the publisher. For information contact Designbase Publishing, 122 East Main Street, Durham, North Carolina 27701.

This book is intended to provide accurate information according to present understanding of the subject matter. It is not intended to be a substitute for the medical advice of physicians. The reader should consult a physician in matters related to HIV/AIDS or other aspects of his health, particularly in respect to any symptoms that may require diagnosis or medical attention.

Library of Congress Cataloging in Publication Data

Faison, Brenda Smith,
  The AIDS handbook.

  Bibliography: p.
  Includes index.
  1. AIDS (Disease) — Popular works. I. Title.
[DNLM: 1. Acquired Immunodeficiency Syndrome—handbooks, manuals, etc.
WD 301 M4738a]
RC607.A26M394   1991   616.97′92   89-25969
ISBN 0-9624040-0-4

Printed in the United States of America

Acknowledgements

Thanks to my many supporters for the contribution they have made to this work. Without their drive and encouragement, I wouldn't have been inspired to probe so many areas.

A special expression of gratitude goes to my editors, Dr. Laila Moustafa, Ph.D., whose editorial suggestions showed remarkable sensitivity and depth of knowledge, and Josh Fraimow, who helped us keep it comprehensive, simple and functional. Also, I would also like to recognize Beverly B. Thompson and Gilbert W. Faison, Jr., for their interviewing and information gathering efforts.

Additionally, I wish to acknowledge the individuals, organizations, agencies and companies who offered ideas and information.

Last, but certainly not least, I appreciate the support and inspiration of my husband, Gilbert W. Faison, Sr., whose idea it was to come up with a handbook on AIDS that would address and speak to all people.

This book is dedicated to those who battle HIV infection/AIDS through personal experience, treatment, care-giving, counseling, funding, research and development, education, and the heightening of awareness.

Table of Contents

Figures and Tables

Introduction

The AIDS Handbook was developed as a comprehensive reference document on AIDS and the AIDS virus. In the past, both federal and private AIDS help organizations have produced individual pamphlets and brochures focusing on individual aspects of AIDS—its effect on men, women or children; concerns about jobs or drug abuse, etc.

This handbook consolidates and simplifies much of that literature, creating one source of information on the basic facts about the disease.

Today, it is absolutely essential that we, the general public, learn all we can about AIDS. The information in this handbook should be responsibly discussed with family members, friends, classmates, co-workers and colleagues.

Until there is a cure for AIDS, education can create a barrier against it. We can stabilize the spread of HIV infection by learning what it is, how it is spread and how it is not spread. Knowing and teaching the facts will eliminate not only the spread of the HIV, but also misconceptions and fear.

1/What AIDS Is

What is HIV Infection?

HIV stands for Human Immunodeficiency Virus. HIV and the AIDS virus are one and the same, and can be used interchangeably. The virus is passed through body fluids such as vaginal secretions, semen and blood. Once you become infected with the HIV, you can spread it to others. The virus primarily causes sickness by making the body unable to fight certain diseases and infections.

WHAT is AIDS?

As defined by the Centers for Disease Control: Acquired Immunodeficiency Syndrome (AIDS) is a specific group of diseases or conditions which are indicative of severe immunosuppression related to infection with the human immunodeficiency virus (HIV).

AIDS is a disease for which there no cure. Another way to think of AIDS for a clearer understanding is:

A	:	**Acquired**	You are not born with it.
I	:	**Immune**	Your body's immune or defense system.
D	:	**Deficiency**	Not working correctly.
S	:	**Syndrome**	A group of signs and symptoms.

AIDS is caused by the Human Immunodeficiency Virus (HIV), which leaves your immune system extremely vulnerable to certain diseases and infections. Again, under normal circumstances, your body would easily ward off such infections. These infections are called "opportunistic" because they take advantage of your weakened immune system in order to invade to the body.

It is these opportunistic diseases and infections that usually kill people with AIDS. However, the HIV can cause two other progressive conditions that are seriously debilitating and eventually cause death—*HIV Encephalopathy* (when the HIV invades the brain causing dementia) and *HIV Wasting Disease*, characterized by serious loss of weight.

What are the Symptoms?

Recent studies show that the AIDS virus (HIV) can lie dormant in your body for a period ranging from 6 months to 7–10 or more years, during which time there may be no symptoms at all. This is known as the incubation period. In fact, fewer than half of the people who have the AIDS virus have any symptoms at all.

Later some infected people may develop severe or prolonged symptoms such as:

- Tiredness (with no clear reason)
- Diarrhea (with no clear reason)
- Fever or Night sweats (which last for several weeks)
- Swollen neck, armpit or groin glands
- White spots or coating on tongue (known as thrush, and may be accompanied by a sore throat)
- Weight loss, greater than 10 lbs., without being on a diet
- Dry coughs, not caused by a cold, flu or smoking
- Pink, blue or purple blotches on or under the skin, inside mouth, nose, eyelids or rectum. These may look like bruises but don't go away. (More common in men than women with AIDS)

Be Aware:

You may have one or more of these signs and not have the AIDS virus. Always check with a medical doctor when you have any of the above signs.

Once an infected person develops AIDS, they may have illnesses that healthy people usually resist. Also, motor and/or memory difficulties, wasting syndrome and a general weakening of body functions may occur.

There are two primary opportunistic diseases that afflict the majority of people who have advanced stages of AIDS. These people can come down with one or both of these diseases: *Kaposi's Sarcoma*, a rare type of cancer that manifests itself through purplish or brown blotches on the skin, mouth or digestive tract; and *Pneumocystis Carinii Pneumonia*, a parasitic infection of the lungs.

How is the HIV Transmitted?

You can't just look at someone and tell whether or not he or she has the AIDS virus. So it's important to know the facts about how the deadly virus is transmitted. HIV is transmitted (spread) through blood-to-blood or sexual contact with someone who has the virus.

You can get the HIV through contact with any body fluid, such as blood, semen, urine, feces, saliva and women's genital secretion. These contacts are usually sexual, and include vaginal, anal and oral intercourse; or the result of blood- to-blood contact, through injecting drugs with needles that have been used by another person. You cannot get the HIV through casual contact such as a hug or handshake. Neither is it spread through the air or in water.

You Can Get the HIV if:

- You have sex with someone who may have HIV/AIDS.
- You inject drugs and share needles with other people.
- You were a baby born of an HIV-infected mother
- You receive blood, blood components or products, or transplants infected with the virus. (very rarely since testing began in 1985)
- You use sperm from an infected donor for artificial insemination (licensed sperm banks screen donors to prevent HIV infection and AIDS).

Table 1 Projected numbers of AIDS cases, deaths attributable to AIDS, and living persons with AIDS, after adjustments for underreporting[1] — United States, 1989–1993

	AIDS Cases		
Year	New Cases[2]	Alive[3]	Deaths
1989	44,000–50,000	92,000–98,000	31,000–34,000
1990	52,000–57,000	101,000–122,000	37,000–42,000
1991	56,000–71,000	127,000–153,000	43,000–52,000
1992	58,000–85,000	139,000–188,000	49,000–64,000
1993	61,000–98,000	151,000–225,000	53,000–76,000
Through 1993[4]	390,000–480,000		285,000–340,000

[1]Projections are adjusted for unreported diagnoses of AIDS by adding 18% to projections obtained from reported cases (corresponding to 85% of all diagnosed cases being reported: 1/0.85 = 1.18) and rounded to the nearest 1000.
[2]Number of cases diagnosed during the year.
[3]Persons with AIDS alive during the year.
[4]Rounded to the nearest 5000. Includes an estimated 120,000 AIDS cases diagnosed through 1988, 48,000 persons with AIDS at the end of 1988, and 72,000 deaths in diagnosed patients through 1988.

Source: Centers for Disease Control, MMWR, Morbidity and Mortality Report, 1990/Vol. 39/No. 7

Questions and Answers About Transmission

Anal sex and sharing needles when injecting drugs can expose you to the AIDS virus.

Q: But what if you have sex with someone other than your regular partner without using a condom?

A: It's risky, plain and simple. Think of it as having sex with everyone with whom your partner has had sex.

Q: But what if you perform fellatio or cunnilingus, or oral sex, on someone?

A: Again, you put yourself at risk. If the receptive partner is infected, then the active partner who performs oral sex can be infected through the partner's semen or vaginal fluid, if a small cut in the mouth, inner cheek or tongue is present. The case is the same if the active partner is infected.

Who Gets AIDS?

As of April 1990, adults and adolescents (13-19 years old) accounted for 130,252 cases of HIV/AIDS reported to the Centers for Disease Control (CDC). There were 118,016 male and 12,236 female. Children under 13 years old accounted for 2,258 cases. These statistics show that the possibility of AIDS striking any member of our population is very real.

Figure 1. How the AIDS Virus Attacks

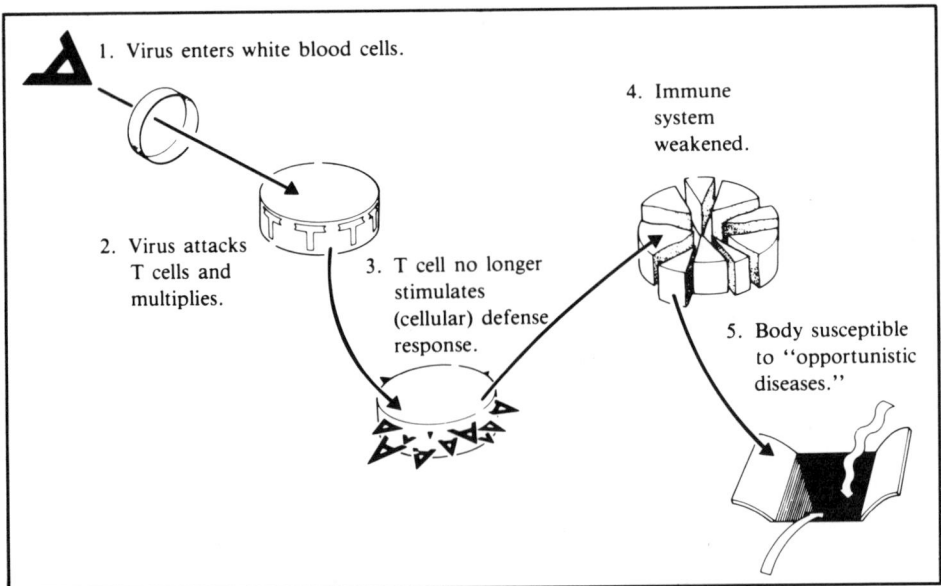

1. Virus enters white blood cells.
2. Virus attacks T cells and multiplies.
3. T cell no longer stimulates (cellular) defense response.
4. Immune system weakened.
5. Body susceptible to "opportunistic diseases."

Source: Surgeon General's Report on Acquired Immunodeficiency Syndrome, U.S. Department of Health and Human Services

Figure 2. Percentages of AIDS Cases by Category (adult male and female).

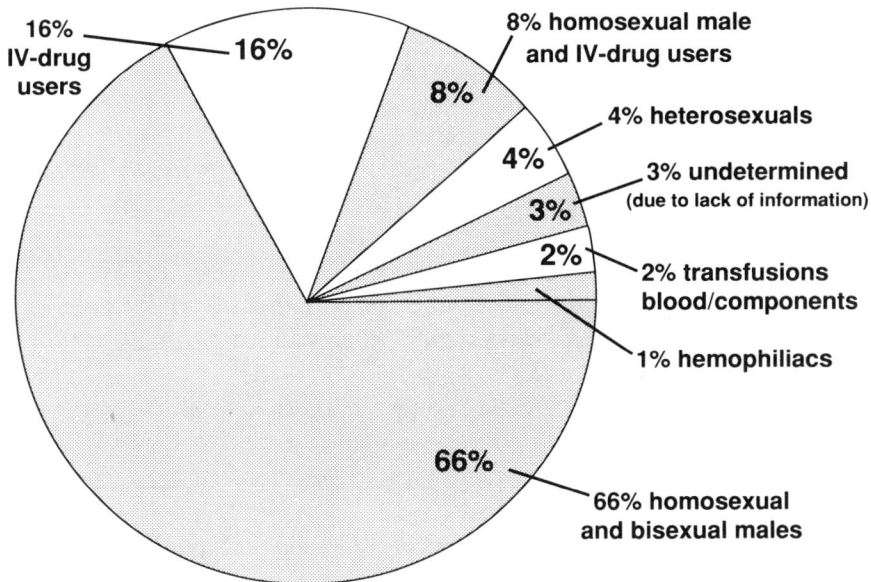

- 16% IV-drug users
- 16%
- 8% homosexual male and IV-drug users
- 8%
- 4% heterosexuals
- 4%
- 3% undetermined (due to lack of information)
- 3%
- 2%
- 2% transfusions blood/components
- 1% hemophiliacs
- 66%
- 66% homosexual and bisexual males

Source: The American Red Cross, Durham County Chapter, N.C.

Figure 3. AIDS Annual Rates per 100,000 Population, for Cases Reported: May 1989 through April 1990, United States

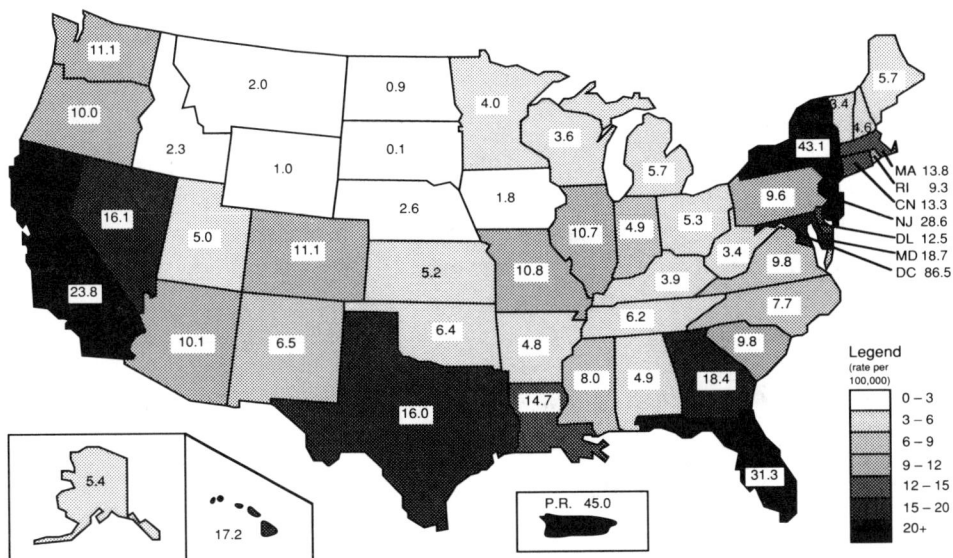

MA 13.8
RI   9.3
CN 13.3
NJ 28.6
DL 12.5
MD 18.7
DC 86.5

Legend (rate per 100,000)
- 0 – 3
- 3 – 6
- 6 – 9
- 9 – 12
- 12 – 15
- 15 – 20
- 20+

P.R. 45.0

Source: HIV/AIDS Surveillance, U.S. Department of Health and Human Services

2/Testing for HIV Antibodies

The only way to find out if you or your partner has the HIV is through testing.

The U.S. Public Health Service Recommends Testing if:

- Since 1977, you have had any sexually transmitted disease.
- You have shared needles, syringes, or other equipment used for injecting drugs.
- You are a man who has had sex with another man.
- You are a prostitute or have had sex with a prostitute, female or male.
- You have had sex with anyone whom you know has done any of the above.
- You are a woman who has engaged in risky behavior and plan to have a baby.
- You are a woman who has engaged in risky behavior and who is not using condoms along with a spermicide as a birth control method.

Your Doctor May Advise You to be Tested if:

- You have hemophilia or have received a blood transfusion, tissue or organ transplant or artificial insemination between 1977 and 1985.

Be Aware:

People who have always practiced safe behavior do not need to be tested. The AIDS antibody test is very reliable if performed by a good laboratory and the results are interpreted by a physician or counselor.

If you have engaged in risky behavior, talk to an AIDS counselor or a doctor who understands AIDS problems.

What to do Before Being Tested

- You should have access to counseling about the test and what the results mean.
- You should be assured that only you and someone you choose will have access to the results of the test.
- Follow-up counseling should be offered whether you test positive or negative.

Types of Tests

There are basically two types of tests.

1. The ELISA Test

The ELISA test detects antibodies to the HIV, the virus that causes AIDS. ELISA is also sometimes called EIA. Both stand for Enzyme-Linked Immunosorbent Assay. This is the test used to screen all donated blood and plasma in the USA (99% accurate). It is also the first test used at clinics, counseling and testing centers, and hospitals.

A positive ELISA test does not mean that you have AIDS now. The test cannot tell if or when you will develop AIDS.

2. The Western Blot Test and IRA

A repeated positive ELIZA test is confirmed by other tests. There are two other tests, the Western Blot and the IRA (Immunofluorescence and Radioimmunoprecipitation Assays), which can be used to confirm a positive ELISA test.

A negative result on one of these tests may not guarantee that you are not infected with the HIV. If you've been infected with the virus recently, a negative test may mean that your body has not had time to develop antibodies against HIV infection. Talk to your healthcare provider about the possibility of further testing.

As it stands now, once you are infected, you will probably be infected for life. But it could take several years for you to start showing symptoms of AIDS.

If you are concerned that you may have been infected, find out about AIDS testing. It can end needless worry.

The Cost of Testing

At your local health department, testing is free; and it can be done anonymously (you do not have to give your name), and you can also receive counseling about whether to be tested or not.

Testing costs vary. Some clinics also offer free testing. However, the fees can range from $20.00 to $100.00 or more. These costs cover retesting required after an initial positive test.

Where to Go to be Tested

Call the National AIDS Hotline (1-800-342-AIDS), your local Red Cross or health department to find out where you can go in your area to get counseling and the HIV test. You can be tested at the following places:

- Your doctor's office
- Hospitals
- Public Health Departments
- Community Laboratories
- Special HIV Testing Centers (in large cities)

Where Not to Go to be Tested

- Never donate blood to the American Red Cross and/or other blood banks and plasma centers as a way of testing for the HIV.
  - This system is already overloaded.
  - This may endanger others if yours is one of the extremely rare cases that escapes detection because of false negative test results.
  - This does not allow for proper counseling before results are given.

What Happens When You Go to Take the Test:

1. You should receive HIV/AIDS counseling both before the test and while waiting for the results.

2. A small amount of blood will be drawn from your arm.

3. The blood will then be taken into a laboratory and analyzed for antibodies to the HIV.

Test Results

You should ask the doctor or counselor about how you will be informed of the test results. Regardless of what the results of your test are, you should request counseling, so that you can better understand what the results of the test mean to you.

If the Results are Positive (HIV-Infected)

- You can infect other people through the exchange of your body fluids.
- You may also infect your unborn child.
- Contact your sexual partner(s) and those you share needles and syringes with, and tell them about the infection.
- Do not share IV drug needles and syringes.
- Get professional counseling to assist you in coping with the realities of your test result.
- Do not donate blood, plasma, body organs, tissue, or semen (sperm).

If The Results Are Negative
- Even though your test may be negative, you may still be infected with the HIV, the virus that causes AIDS. Why? Because HIV antibodies may not have yet developed.
- You should continue to take precautions to protect yourself and your partner from this point on.
- Through further counseling, you may find that other tests are needed.

The Right To Anonymity
In many cases, you will want the results of your test to be kept private, There are two ways to do this:

1. If the test is "**confidential,**" the results will be available to a limited number of medical personnel. Ask your counselor or doctor how the results will be filed.

2. You may ask for an "**anonymous**" test if you want the results to be even more private. With anonymous testing your results cannot be traced to you. In most cases all test information and results are numbered, and you are the only one who knows the number which is assigned to your test.

An Excerpt From the Surgeon General's Report on AIDS, Concerning the Right to Know
"Because there is no vaccine to prevent AIDS, and no cure, many feel there is nothing to be gained by revealing sexual contacts that might also be infected with the AIDS virus. When a community or state requires reporting of those infected with the AIDS virus to public health authorities in order to trace sexual and intravenous drug contacts—as is the practice with other sexually transmitted diseases—those infected with the AIDS virus go underground out of the mainstream of health care and education. For this reason, current public health practice is to protect the privacy of the individual infected with the AIDS virus and to maintain the strictest confidentiality concerning his/her health records."

Be Aware:
If you would like to know more about AIDS and your HIV test, talk to your doctor, local health department, or hospital. For more information, see "Information, Counseling and Support."

Table 2   Number and percentage of HIV-antibody tests and positive tests at publicly funded sites reported to CDC, by type of test site—United States, January 1988–September 1989.

Test site	No. Tested	HIV Positive No.	HIV Positive (%)	Total Tests (%)	Total HIV positive (%)
Freestanding site	562,647	32,440	(5.8)	(40.1)	(50.4)
Sexually transmitted diseases clinic	353,643	11,985	(3.4)	(25.2)	(18.6)
Private physician's office/ clinic	84,752	2,927	(3.5)	(6.0)	(4.6)
Family-planning clinic	65,838	450	(0.7)	(4.7)	(0.7)
Prison	55,853	3,538	(6.3)	(4.0)	(5.5)
Prenatal/obstetric clinic	47,834	382	(0.8)	(3.4)	(0.6)
Other public health department	36,198	3,266	(9.0)	(2.6)	(5.1)
Drug-treatment center	18,632	1,004	(5.4)	(1.3)	(1.6)
College	14,738	610	(4.1)	(1.1)	(1.0)
Tuberculosis clinic	10,974	458	(4.2)	(0.8)	(0.7)
Other nonhealth department sites	108,340	4,540	(4.2)	(7.7)	(7.1)
Unclassified sites	43,791	2,747	(6.3)	(3.1)	(4.3)
Total	**1,403,240**	**64,347**	**(4.6)**	**(100.0)**	**(100.0)**

Source: Centers for Disease Control (CDC) Morbidity and Mortality Weekly Reports (MMWR) 1990/Vol. 39/No. 9.

Talking to Your Partner About HIV/AIDS

The good news about HIV/AIDS is that it can be prevented. Once you know the facts, there is no reason why you can not enjoy safe sex. Both you and your partner are responsible for protection against HIV infection. Your partner is probably as concerned about staying healthy as you are. You should both study, learn more and share the facts.

Things to Keep in Mind When Talking with Your Sexual Partner:

- Discuss protection with your partner before intercourse takes place. Plan a time to talk about it before you or your partner are in a sexual mood, and have the talk outside of your bedroom.
- It is your right to ask questions about your partner's past. If you are concerned about the answers, or if he or she does not want to take precautions, you may choose not to have sex with that person.
- A show of concern means that you care and are interested in the health and safety of your partner, and yourself; it does not mean you don't trust him or her.
- If you have any doubts about the faithfulness of your present partner, or the safety of your own past sexual behavior since 1977, then testing for the HIV (the AIDS virus) is suggested for you and your partner. HIV/AIDS counseling is also recommended. Don't take chances with each other's health and life.
- If your relationship is violent or abusive, it may be difficult to talk about protection with your partner, because sensitive subjects like AIDS or using protection may create more negative feelings.
- Get help from a counselor or someone else who can assist with relationship problems if you can't have this type of discussion without having a fight. Organizations and shelters for battered or abused women can be found through your local health department or your local yellow pages directory.

Safe, Low-risk and High-risk Behavior

In order to stop the spread of the HIV (the AIDS virus), it is necessary to know what behavior puts you at risk of HIV infection. Most high-risk factors center around sex and drug use.

Below is a list of behaviors in three categories, "Safe Behavior", "Low-risk behavior" and "High-risk Behavior."

Safe Behavior

- Abstinence or celibacy
- Sex with no physical contact
- Oral, anal or vaginal intercourse, with a partner who you know is HIV-free (through testing) in a relationship in which both are monogamous, and
- Not participating in any form of drug abuse; this includes alcohol
- Using new and disposable needles and syringes each time, if injecting drugs; prescribed and non-prescribed
- Other forms of intimacy (such as body rubs) which do not involve an exchange of body fluids
- Sex toys, not shared
- Hugging

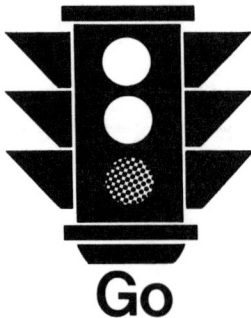

Low-risk Behavior

- All types of sex; oral, anal, or vaginal, using a latex condom and a spermicide (nonoxynol-9) with any person whose HIV/AIDS status you are not sure of
- Sex with an HIV/AIDS-infected partner, using a latex glove for masturbation, fingering, etc.

Note:

- Never use a spermicide without a condom
- Though the condom (or latex glove) and spermicide further reduce the risk of infection, they still do not totally eliminate the risk of transmission of the HIV
- Cleaning used syringes with bleach and water in order to share or reuse. (Risk is introduced when the user is careless in the cleaning process)
- Allowing yourself to be tattooed. (tattoo artists may not use clean needles between each use)
- French kissing (deep or open mouth kissing) with an infected person

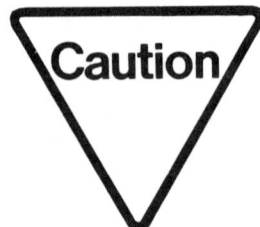

Go

Caution

High-risk Behavior

- Sex with an HIV-infected partner **without** using a condom, spermicide and latex glove. This includes vaginal, anal and oral sex, as well as fingering, fisting, etc.
- Sex with a partner who has engaged and/or engages in anal sex
- Sex with a prostitute, male or female, or anyone who is promiscuous
- Sharing sex toys
- Sex with an intravenous drug abuser
- Injecting drugs with needles and syringes that have been used by others
- Sex with natural membrane condoms such as lambskin (Only use latex condoms.)
- Watersports in mouth
- Using a spermicide without a condom

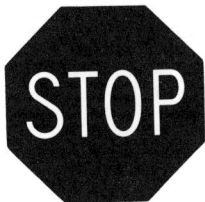

STOP

Is the Use of A Condom With a Spermicide a Good Idea?

Yes.

In lab test studies, nonoxynol-9, the active ingredient in spermicides, has been shown to make the HIV inactive. Latex condoms provide greater protection when used with a water-based contraceptive (birth control) foam.

Using both condom and spermicide provides an optimum low-risk environment. However, this combination still does not provide total protection. (see "Why Do Condoms Fail" in this chapter.)

Spermicide (nonoxynol-9) Is Found In:

- Contraceptive (birth control) foams
- Gels
- Creams
- Suppositories
- Some lubricants
- Some lubricated condoms
- Contraceptive sponges

Be Aware:

- Never use a spermicide alone instead of a condom.
- Both the spermicide and condom should be in place **before** foreplay, genital contact or penetration occurs.
- If a lubricant is used, be sure that it is **water-based.** Do not use oil-based lubricants! Oil-based lubricants, such as those made with mineral oil petroleum jelly, vegetable oil, or cold cream, may damage the condom.
- Always use a new condom each time you have intercourse or oral sex. **Before** foreplay, genital contact or penetration, place a new condom on the penis. Keep in mind that contact with **any body fluid** can cause contact with the AIDS virus or other sexually transmitted disease (STD) organisms.

Table 3 **Reported use of latex condoms** during the 6 months before interview by 16,998 intravenous-drug users not in drug treatment — selected sites, 1987–1989

Gender/Sexual Behavior	No. respondents[1]	Use of condoms		
		Always	Sometimes	Never
Men				
Vaginal insertive	10,270	10%	20%	70%
Oral insertive	7,128	8%	7%	85%
Oral receptive	283	18%	19%	63%
Anal insertive	2,469	13%	14%	73%
Homosexual/Bisexual	404	20%	28%	53%
Heterosexual	2,065	11%	11%	78%
Anal receptive	234	29%	23%	48%
Women				
Vaginal receptive	3,635	14%	29%	57%
Oral receptive	2,403	15%	19%	66%
Anal receptive	566	16%	16%	68%

[1]Respondents may practive more than one type of sexual behavior and are thus counted in each appropriate sexual-behavior category.

Source: Centers for Disease Control, Morbidity and Mortality Weekly Report (MMWR) 1990/Vol. 39/No. 16.

Instructions for the Use of a Condom and Spermicide

1. Apply the spermicide. Use the manufacturer's suggested instructions and application device (where required). Instructions will vary from one type and brand to another.

2. In putting on the condom, pull it over the head of the erect penis. To avoid an air pocket, squeeze reservoir end (tip of condom) slightly to release air.

3. Slowly unroll the condom **all the way to the base of the penis.** If the condom does not unroll all the way to the base, it has been put on incorrectly and should be removed and thrown away. Use a new one.

4. As soon as possible after ejaculation, climax or "coming," **hold the rim of the condom against the penis and withdraw** the penis slowly, while it is still somewhat erect.

5. During this time, keep the penis well away from your partner's body. Be sure to **hold the top of the condom** (the rim) **firmly when withdrawing,** to avoid spilling the semen.

6. Remove the condom, **discard** it, and **wash** hands and genital area.

Figure 4. How to Use a Condom.

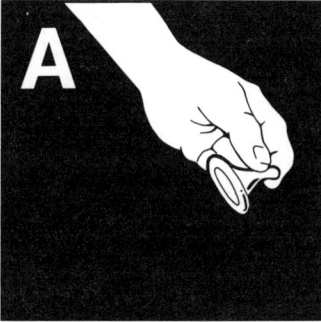

Hold tip of condom to squeeze out air. Place condom on end of erect penis.

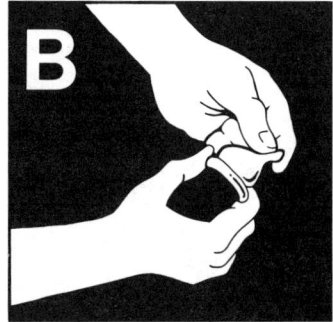

Keep holding tip of condom while slowly unrolling the condom on head of penis.

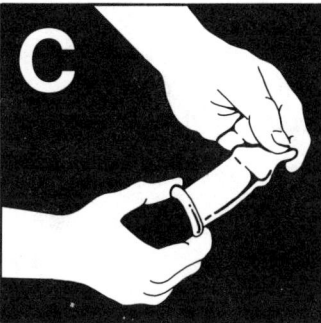

Continue unrolling the condom down to the base of penis.

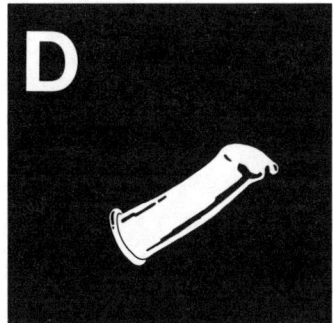

When rim of condom reaches base (touching pubic hair) of the penis it has been put on correctly.

Be Aware:

- If for any reason semen spills out or leaks out during use, or if the condom breaks, both partners should clean themselves wherever contact may have occurred, as soon as possible.
- Wash the hands, penis and surrounding area immediately before and after sexual contact. This will further reduce the chance of HIV infection.
- Condoms should be stored in a cool, dry place. Do not store condoms in your back pocket, glove compartment or anyplace warm. Heat can weaken the material and cause tears or holes in the condom during sex.
- Carefully inspect the condom. If the rubber material is brittle, sticky or obviously damaged, do not use it.
- Condoms can be used for oral sex on men.

Why Condoms Fail and What You Can Do to Prevent Failure

Studies show that the failure rate of condoms as a birth control device is about 10 percent. Because the price of failure may mean contracting a disease that can cause death, this 10 percent failure rate cannot be ignored. Knowing why condoms fail will increase your success rate when using them.

Why condoms fail:

- Because "people are only human," often condoms are not used **when** they should be.
- Condoms are often used too late. They should be applied **before** any genital contact takes place. Remember pre- ejaculatory fluid, vaginal secretions and other body fluids can contain the HIV.
- Condoms are often put on incorrectly and are sometimes left on too long. Follow instructions carefully.
- Very rarely, condoms may have a manufacturing defect which may cause tearing and breaking. Use only U.S. manufactured condoms, which are monitored for quality control.
- Some people use natural skin condoms like lambskin, instead of latex condoms. **Only use latex condoms.** Natural skin condoms contain tiny pores which can allow the HIV to pass through and also tear more easily than latex condoms.

Will Condoms Change Sex For You?

The use of condoms can protect you from, and reduce your fear of, getting the HIV and other sexually transmitted diseases. With a little imagination, low-risk protection can become a part of your sexual experience.

At first, you and your partner may find that using condoms feel a little different. But don't give up. Practice makes perfect, and it's possible to adapt quickly to this new sensation—particularly with an accepting partner.

You should make putting on the condom part of your lovemaking. Be sure the condom goes on before the penis has contact with the mouth, vagina or anus.

Where to Purchase Condoms and Other Protection

Condoms, foams and lubricants can be purchased at:

- Your local drug store.
- Your local health clinic.
- Grocery stores.
- Convenience stores.
- Some public rest rooms.
- Direct from catalogs (condoms).

Be Aware:

Be sure to use U.S. manufactured condoms, which are tested for quality control.

About Making Excuses

In 1989 studies showed that more high-risk men were practicing safe sex, while only a few were still having unsafe sex. By the first quarter of 1990, however, this achievement was reversing. Sadly, many men were "slipping" and losing sight of the seriousness and ease of transmission of the HIV. Unsafe sex must be completely eliminated among all sexually active persons in order to stop the spread of the AIDS virus.

When considering sex without protection; remember:

- Occasional unsafe sex or "slipping" ignores the deadly consequences of AIDS. With just one slip you can easily become infected, or infect someone else.
- Being in love or a long-time association does not make you immune to AIDS. Unless you are certain that both of you have been monogamous and are free of the virus, you **must** have safe sex. Otherwise, you may give the HIV to or get it from, your partner.
- None of the reasons for not using condoms outweigh the fact that they

reduce the spread of HIV infection. Get beyond the excuses, and **always protect yourself.** Use a latex condom with a spermicide containing nonoxynol-9.

- If you are creative and use your imagination, safe sex need never be boring, but fun and enjoyable.
- No one is immune to HIV/AIDS. If you have been having unsafe sex and have not yet been infected, don't think you're immune. You've just been lucky. Start practicing safe sex!
- Some HIV-infected persons, or those who think they are infected, assume that safe sex no longer matters. They are wrong. You can infect someone else, and repeated exposure to the HIV makes you more likely to develop AIDS.
- If you have been having unsafe sex, STOP NOW! HIV/AIDS prevention means **always** using condoms and **never** sharing needles and syringes.

Cleaning Used Needles and Syringes

If you don't have access to disposable needles and syringes you should know how to properly clean used ones.

Figure 5. How to Clean Used Needles and Syringes   **Source:** SFAF

1. BLEACH

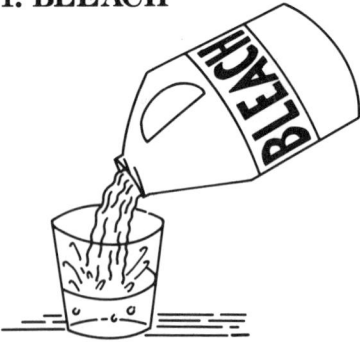

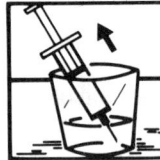

A. Fill Syringe   B. Empty Syringe

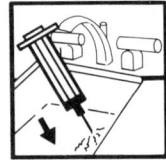

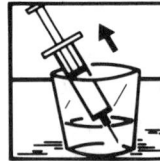

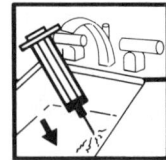

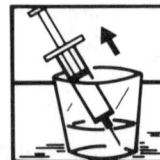

C. Fill Syringe   D. Empty Syringe

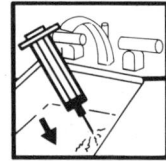

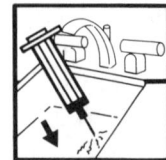

2. WATER   Note: Be sure not to shoot or drink the bleach.

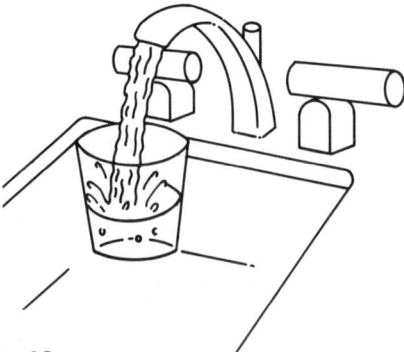

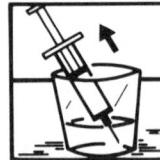

A. Fill Syringe   B. Empty Syringe

C. Fill Syringe   D. Empty Syringe

Be Aware:

- When the use of such an injection device is required, use prepackaged, sanitized, disposable needles and syringes.
- All intravenous drug users should be aware of the risk factor involved in spreading HIV infection and should know how to clean used syringes and needles effectively.
- Do not shoot or drink the bleach.

How to Dispose of Used Needles and Syringes.

Outside of the Healthcare Setting:

1. To reduce chances of sticking yourself during disposal, place point of the needle on a hard surface, such as a table top, floor or street surface (concrete).

- Push the needle into the surface enough to bend the point of the needle under.

2. Replace plastic cap over needle and place in plastic bag and discard.

Inside the Healthcare Setting:

1. Never recap needles before throwing them away (this is a major cause of puncture injury).

2. Place them in a puncture-resistant plastic container used only for this purpose.

Table 4   Percentage of 16,998 intravenous-drug users not in drug treatment who reported using new drug-injection equipment or cleaning used equipment during the 6 months before interview — selected sites, 1987–1989

Behavior	No. respondents	Frequency					
		Always	>50% time	50% time	<50% time	Never	Unknown
Used new needle	16,998	20%	38%	20%	18%	3%	1%
Cleaned needle[1]	13,528[2]	63%	14%	8%	8%	6%	1%
Used bleach[3]	12,679[4]	14%	16%	11%	20%	38%	2%

[1]Respondents could report cleaning needles by any of several methods and still be consistent with an "always" response.
[2]Excludes those who reported always using a new needle.
[3]A subset of those who cleaned needles.
[4]Excludes those who reported never cleaning their drug-injection equipment.

Source: Centers for Disease Control, Morbidity and Mortality Weekly Report (MMWR) 1990/Vol. 39/No. 16.

4/The Effect of AIDS on Your Job

For workers in general, there is no need for worry or special precautions when it comes to working with an HIV-infected person. A fellow employee who has AIDS or who carries the HIV (the AIDS virus) does not endanger you. The AIDS virus in not spread in the air you breath or the food you eat; nor is it spread by routine, nonsexual, everyday contact.

The following are guidelines and answers to some questions which may arise for workers in certain occupations:

Should People With AIDS be Allowed to Work?

People diagnosed with HIV/AIDS pose no risk to their co-workers, the public or themselves. They should be able to work as long as they feel well enough to do so.

Many companies that have had experience in dealing with employees with AIDS have determined that it can be handled as any other life-threatening illness, such as heart disease and cancer. Thousands of people who have been diagnosed with HIV/AIDS remain gainfully employed.

What about Food Service Workers?

The HIV (the AIDS virus) is not transmitted in food, so people who work with food, such as cooks, caterers, bartenders, waiters, airline attendants and others, should not be restricted from work because they have been infected with the HIV.

All food service workers should certainly observe good personal hygiene and sanitary food handling methods. This also includes those with the HIV. While preparing food, workers should take particular care to avoid injury to their hands.

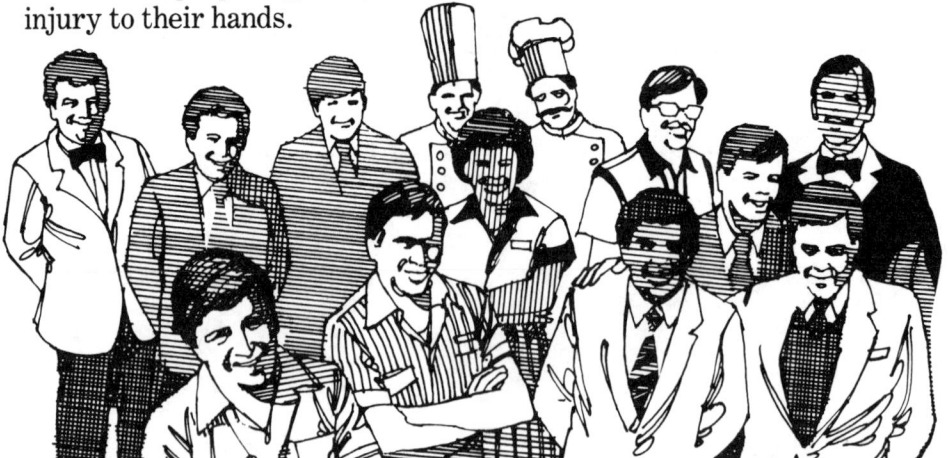

How Can Personal Service Workers Protect Themselves?

Personal service workers include beauticians, barbers, cosmetologists, electrologists, and manicurists. People working in these fields systematically observe procedures that protect them and their clients from bacterial and viral infections. When instruments that could draw blood are used, it is important to use sterilizing equipment, though the risk of spreading the HIV in this setting is minimal.

The following are some guidelines:

- Skin-penetrating instruments, such as ear-piercing devices and needles used for electrolysis, acupuncture and tattooing, should be either discarded after one use, or thoroughly cleaned and disinfected between uses with a chemical germicide.

- The same procedure should be followed for other sharp instruments, such as razors or cuticle scissors.

- A personal service worker should not make direct contact with open or weeping sores until the wound has healed.

How Can Special Precaution Job Workers Avoid Infection?

Workers with jobs requiring special precautions, such as police personnel, firefighters, emergency medical workers and prison employees, could be exposed to blood or other body fluids of people with HIV/AIDS or HIV-related disorders. This exposure can be caused through accidents, fires or violence. Fortunately, workers can avoid infection by following a few simple rules:

- Be Aware. Avoid punctures and wounds from hypodermic needles used by drug abusers or as weapons. The blood on these items could cause HIV infection.

- When handling contaminated items, always use disposable gloves. Put contaminated items in a cut-proof evidence bag to be delivered to a laboratory for examination or disposal.

- Use freshly diluted household bleach to clean up blood spills promptly. (one part bleach to 10 parts water).

- If mouth-to-mouth resuscitation is necessary for a person with HIV/AIDS, use an "S-tube" or a hand-operated resuscitator bag.

- Because hand washing reduces the chance of spreading infection, wash your hands after exposure to any possible source of infection.

- If there is a chance of exposure to the blood or any other body fluids of someone with AIDS, wear protective masks, gowns, gloves and shoe coverings.

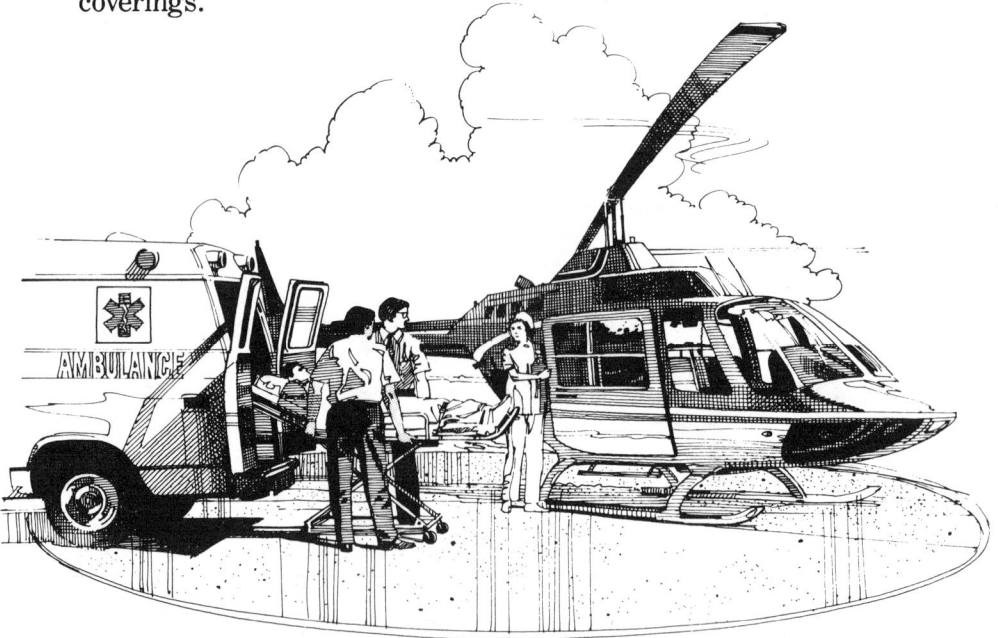

Where to Find Other Specific Special Precaution Job Information:

The American Red Cross offers free brochures on HIV/AIDS and specific professions. These are available through local Red Cross chapters:

"Your Job and AIDS: Are there risks?" Stock # 329502

"Emergency and Public Safety Workers and HIV/AIDS—A Duty to Respond." Stock # 329544.

"HIV Infection and Workers in Health Care Settings." Stock # 329545.

"A Guide to Home Care for the Person with AIDS." Stock # 329542.

"School Systems and AIDS: Information for Teachers and School Officials." Stock # 329541.

"Children and AIDS, Information for Teachers and School Officials." Stock # 329505.

For More Information on HIV/AIDS in the Workplace:

- Ask your employee representatives—supervisor, manager, union representative or personnel department—to keep informed about HIV/AIDS, and to keep you and your co-workers informed.

- Other Sources Include:
  - Your doctor
  - Your state or local health department
  - The Public Health Service's AIDS Hotline
    Toll free: 1-800-342-AIDS
  - The American Red Cross (local chapter)

5/The Safety of the Blood Supply

Since March 1985 all donated blood and blood products have been tested for the AIDS virus antibody. All units with positive results are discarded.

Today, the risk of getting AIDS from a blood transfusion is minimal. So small, in fact, that no one should ever postpone or cancel non-elective surgery. Statistics indicate that between 1978 and 1984, about 2 percent of all AIDS cases resulted from blood transfusions. The chances of contracting AIDS from a transfusion range from 1 in 40,000 to 1 in 250,000 depending on where the blood was donated.

Donating Blood

You cannot get AIDS from donating blood, plasma or any other blood component. Needles are used only once and then discarded. Because there is no substitute for life-sustaining blood, all healthy adults not at risk for getting AIDS are urged to donate.

Protecting the Blood Supply

In the late 1970s, no one could have guessed the consequences of AIDS for the blood supply. When scientists first learned that the virus could be spread through blood, public health officials urged people who had AIDS symptoms and those known to be at risk for AIDS not to donate.

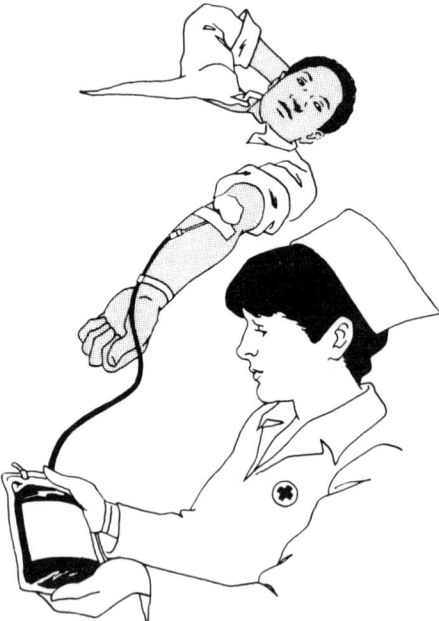

A method of screening donors was developed, and those at risk for HIV infection were not allowed to donate blood. New heat and chemical procedures were developed to kill viruses in clotting factor concentrates, manufactured for use in treating hemophilia.

In 1984, the HIV virus was discovered. This meant that scientists could develop a test to detect antibodies to the virus. Antibodies are proteins that cells make to destroy specific viruses and other germs. Almost a year later, by the spring of 1985, a test to detect the antibody was being used at blood and plasma centers nationwide.

The Accuracy of Tests

The test used to detect the AIDS virus antibody, the ELISA test, is considered highly reliable. However, like all blood tests, it is not 100 percent reliable in identifying infected persons. False positives and false negatives are possible, meaning that blood tests may indicate a non-infected person has the AIDS virus, when he or she actually doesn't, and vice versa. All positive tests are repeated to confirm the results and, then the Western Blot test is done to confirm the ELISA results. In any case, all units of blood that test positive for the AIDS virus are carefully disposed of. (See "Testing for HIV Antibodies").

Today, the risks of refusing a blood transfusion, for surgeries or other emergencies, far outweigh the risks of getting HIV/AIDS from a blood transfusion.

Alternative Sources for Donated Blood

Autologus Donations

Autologus donations, or giving blood for one's own scheduled elective surgery, is recommended in many cases. It is estimated that by 1995, about 20 percent of all donations will be autologous. However, the public is still strongly urged to donate blood to meet the needs of those who cannot donate for themselves.

Directed Donations

Having someone you know donate blood for you is another alternative, referred to as directed donations. However, there is no evidence that directed donations are any safer than donations from the general public. All donations are tested for the AIDS virus antibody, syphilis and hepatitis.

Also, if for some reason the directed donor's blood tests positive, he or she stands to face possible embarrassment from the knowledge that his or her blood cannot be transfused.

6/Drug Abuse and AIDS

Should Drug Abusers be Concerned About AIDS?

Yes.

People who shoot drugs are second in line as the group at greatest risk for AIDS. Homosexual and bisexual men are the most prevalent groups. Many HIV-infected people are heroin, cocaine or speed users who use needles to inject drugs. People who shoot drugs become infected by sharing their paraphernalia (works; i.e., needles, syringes, cookers, cotton, etc.) with HIV-infected people when injecting ("mainlining" or "skin popping") drugs.

After injecting drugs, the smallest amount of blood left in used drug paraphernalia can contain the HIV. Even if the blood cannot be seen in or on these items, the virus can still be present.

Remember, drug abuse has always been dangerous. Now, with the threat of HIV infection/AIDS, it is more dangerous than ever before. Studies show that in some cities, more than half of all IV drug users are HIV-infected, and thousands of them have AIDS. You may already be infected if you and/or your partner have shared needles since 1977.

Who is at Risk Because of the Drug Abuser?

- The spouse and/or sexual partner(s) of the drug user
- The babies of the drug user

What About Poppers?

Poppers is the slang term for a mixture of chemicals used as an inhalant to achieve a "high." They are yet another recreational drug. Poppers are used commonly during social events such as dancing and for muscle relaxation during sex. Poppers are most commonly used in the lesbian and gay population, but have been experimented with by others as well.

The active ingredients in poppers are **amyl and butyl nitrites.** Poppers are not regulated or tested by any government agency.

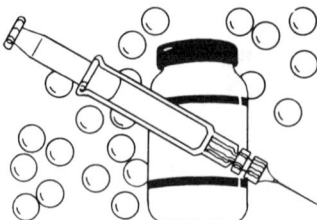

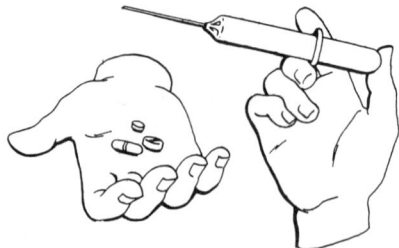

What Can Poppers Do to You?

Researchers have found that the use of poppers:

- Damages the body's ability to stay healthy.
- Leads to specific diseases.
- Is suspected to have played a part in causing AIDS.
- Weakens the body's immune system, which may lead to the development of the cancer *Kaposi's Sarcoma* (KS), one of the diseases linked to AIDS.
- Can cause health problems not related to AIDS, including headaches and dizziness, fainting and even death.
- Interferes with judgement and lessens awareness of the severity of physical acts, which may result in trauma to body organs.
- Makes people more likely to participate in unsafe sex, and places themselves at high risk for exposure to the HIV.

What Does Alcohol Have to do With the Spread of the HIV?

When you are under the influence of alcohol and other drugs, you may do things which you would not do under normal circumstances. You may not think to use the proper protection to prevent HIV infection. So when you are thinking of using alcohol, keep in mind:

- Researchers have found that when people use alcohol and other drugs, they are much less likely to use condoms and other protection measures.
- Alcohol and drugs damage your immune system. If you are HIV-infected, your immune system needs to be as strong as it can be.
- Alcohol and drugs do not cause AIDS, but the use of both can lead to unsafe sex and the sharing of needles, which can in turn lead to infection with the AIDS virus.
- If it is difficult for you to maintain safe sex practices, it may be because of alcohol and drug use.
- Use of alcohol, and other recreational drugs such as marijuana, angel dust or PCP, cocaine, crack, poppers, and others not prescribed by your doctor, increases your chances of becoming HIV-infected.

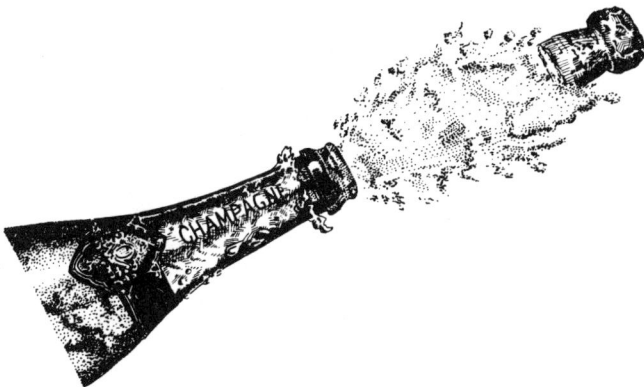

Prevention For All Drug Abusers

- Consider reducing or stopping the use of alcohol and illegal and unregulated drugs in your life. Stopping is the best way to protect yourself and those you love. Don't continue to risk your health.
- Do not share needles, syringes, cookers or works with anyone. If you must share needles and syringes, clean it first with bleach. (See "How to Clean Used Hypodermic Needles and Syringes.")
- Do not rent or buy works that have been used by someone else. Inspect all packages carefully to insure that they have not been tampered with. (Used syringes and needles are sometimes sold as new in resealed packaging.)
- To avoid transmitting the virus further, properly dispose of your works. People may find them laying around and stick themselves.
- Avoid sex with people who have HIV/AIDS. If you do have sex with someone who is infected, use both a condom and spermicide to lower risk of transmission. Avoid body fluids, especially semen and blood. (See "Using A Condom With A Spermicide.")
- Avoid sex practices that may cause injury to body tissue, such as anal sex, and limit yourself to one sex partner.
- See a doctor or visit a clinic for an examination and an HIV antibody test to find out if you may have already been infected with the AIDS virus.
- If learning to refuse poppers or any other chemical substance is a problem, get help. Contact a support group, a drug treatment program or a sex counseling center. (For drug treatment see "Drug Abuse and Alcohol Treatment and Prevention Programs.")
- Keep current on developments in HIV/AIDS research.

Be Aware:

Today, the use of alcohol and other drugs is one of the most common reasons why people become HIV-infected.

7/AIDS and Men

In many cities across America, AIDS is the leading cause of death of young men. HIV/AIDS doesn't care where you live, whether you are heterosexual (straight), homosexual (gay) or bisexual, what ethnic group you belong to or where you work. The HIV does not discriminate. People do not get AIDS because of who they are.

How do Men get AIDS?

1. Transmission through sex

- Unsafe sex (exposure to the body fluids of an HIV-infected person)
- Having sex with infected men or women (oral, anal and/or vaginal sex)
- Sex with well-known and unknown promiscuous partners
- Sharing sex toys

2. Transmission through Sharing Needles and Other Works

- Through IV drug use, sharing drug needles and syringes with an infected person
- Sharing used cotton, cookers, and other items (works) used in IV drug use
- Through blood transfusions or blood products donated by infected persons (before blood donors were carefully screened and tested; this is a very small percentage of the total cases)
- Tattoo needles

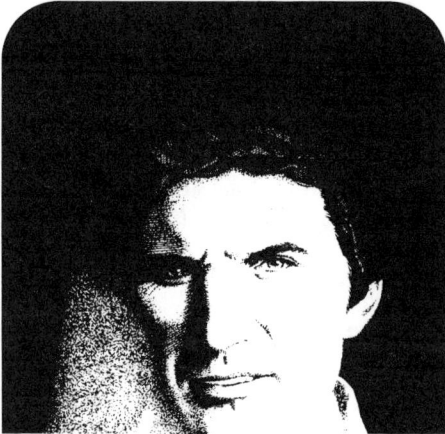

Homosexual and Bisexual Men

Though AIDS is a disease which has effected every group within our society, it is especially prevalent among homosexual and bisexual men. Important changes such as choosing only safe sex and partners with whom you can have safe sex is essential. Because these are actually life or death decisions, you have to learn to say no. Remember, the key to safe sex is that no bodily fluids are exchanged.

Anal Intercourse

If you are involved in anal intercourse, use a condom along with a spermicide. It is during this form of sexual intercourse that the rectal lining can be injured, allowing the HIV and/or other germs to enter the bloodstream. If sex toys (dildos, etc.) are used, don't share and be sure to keep them clean.

Other forms of anal penetration such a fisting and fingering can be means of transmission, again, because of injury to rectal tissue. These can cause the passing of germs to the bloodstream and bowel, while exposing your finger and/or hand to germs and, if tissue injury occurs, to your partner's blood. Fisting is a high-risk activity and **should be avoided**. Fingering may be somewhat safer, provided there is no broken skin. Keep fingernails trimmed close to prevent tissue breaking. Also, a latex glove may be used if your partner's HIV/AIDS status is unknown.

Oral-anal Intercourse

Oral-anal sex (rimming) is high-risk behavior. Here you are exposed to various fecal germs. The receiving partner may absorb saliva into his blood stream. HIV is only one of several infections that you are exposed to through this behavior. **It should be avoided** in order to stay strong and healthy.

Oral-penile Intercourse

In oral stimulation of the penis (sucking) remember that pre-ejaculatory fluid and semen are body fluids that can contain the AIDS virus. Keeping these fluids out of your mouth is the best way to reduce the risk of exposure. A latex condom can be used in oral-penile sex.

Kissing/Hugging

When there are sores or open cuts in either partner's mouth, kissing represents some risk.

Hugging is indeed a safe behavior. Be mindful of the key to safe sex: avoid the exchange of body fluids.

Mutual Masturbation

This form of masturbation (jacking off) is safe, again, as long as semen and/or pre-ejaculatory fluid does not get into a cut on your hand. Latex gloves will lower the risk of HIV infection during this activity. Other forms of bodily contact, such as touching and body rubs, are also safe.

Water Sports

When taking part in water sports (urinating on partner), broken skin and your mouth become points of entry for the HIV. If you participate in water sports, avoid it when broken skin is present and keep your mouth closed.

Be Aware:

As in all forms of sexual activity, thoroughly wash all areas which have contacted any body fluid. Avoid any blood-to-blood contact.

Table 5. Male adult/adolescent AIDS cases by exposure category, and race/ethnicity, reported through April 1990, United States

Male exposure category	White, not Hispanic No.	(%)	Black, not Hispanic No.	(%)	Hispanic No.	(%)	Asian/ Pacific Islander No.	(%)	American Indian/ Alaskan Native No.	(%)	Total[4] No.	(%)
Male homosexual/bisexual contact	56,169	(80)	12,927	(44)	8,257	(47)	600	(81)	90	(62)	78,212	(66)
Intravenous (IV) drug use (heterosexual)	4,268	(6)	10,242	(35)	6,921	(39)	21	(3)	15	(10)	21,530	(18)
Male homosexual/bisexual contact and IV drug use	5,261	(8)	2,349	(8)	1,289	(7)	13	(2)	24	(16)	8,948	(8)
Hemophilia/coagulation disorder	957	(1)	74	(0)	87	(0)	15	(2)	6	(4)	1,143	(1)
Heterosexual contact:	420	(1)	2,030	(7)	217	(1)	6	(1)	1	(1)	2,678	(2)
Sex with IV drug user	270		545		147		1		1		964	
Sex with person with hemophilia	4		1		—		—		—		5	
Born in Pattern-II[1] country	2		1,318		7		3		—		1,333	
Sex with person born in Pattern-II country	24		24		4		—		—		52	
Sex with transfusion recipient with HIV infection	19		9		1		—		—		30	
Sex with HIV-infected person, risk not specified	101		133		58		2		—		294	
Receipt of blood transfusion, blood components, or tissue[2]	1,449	(2)	273	(1)	156	(1)	42	(6)	1	(1)	1,925	(2)
Other/undetermined[3]	1,411	(2)	1,262	(4)	824	(5)	44	(6)	9	(6)	3,580	(3)
Male Total	**69,935**	**(100)**	**29,157**	**(100)**	**17,751**	**(100)**	**741**	**(100)**	**146**	**(100)**	**118,016**	**(100)**

[1] Countries with a distinctive pattern of transmission termed ''Pattern II'' by the World Health Organization.

[2] Includes 8 transfusion recipients who received blood screened by HIV antibody, and 1 tissue recipient.

[3] ''Other'' refers to 2 health-care workers who seroconverted to HIV and developed AIDS after occupational exposure to HIV-infected blood. ''Undetermined'' refers to patients whose mode of exposure to HIV is unknown. This includes patients under investigation; patients who died, were lost to follow-up or refused interview; and patients whose mode of exposure to HIV remains undetermined after investigation.

[4] Includes 2286 males and 30 females whose race ethnicity is unknown.

SOURCE: HIV/AIDS Surveillance U.S. Department of Health and Human Services, 1990.

As the AIDS epidemic grows, an increasing number of women are in danger of getting HIV/AIDS. Currently, more than 8 percent of the people with AIDS are women.

It is vital that women know how to prevent HIV infection, which can lead to AIDS. You can and need to take responsibility for protecting your health. Learn the facts and take action to protect yourself and the people you care about.

How Have Women Become Infected?

- Through IV Drug use
- Having sexual partners who were IV Drug users
- Having sex with partners who became HIV-infected by having sex with other infected men or women
- Through the menstrual blood of another female who was HIV-infected during sexual relations (1 case reported)
- Many women with HIV/AIDS were the sex partners of men who became infected from infected blood transfusions or blood products. (used to treat diseases like hemophilia and used for transfusions), or were themselves infected during blood transfusion before screening guidelines were adopted in 1985. (See "The Safety of the Nation's Blood Supply.")

Be Aware:

It is possible for women to have become infected before, during, and after pregnancy.

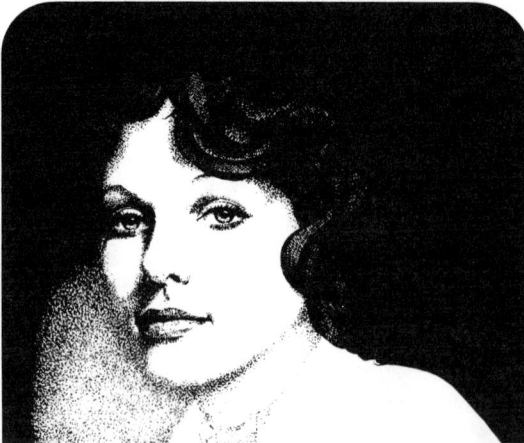

The Safest Protection Is:

- Not having sex.
- Not sharing drug needles or syringes.
- Not shooting drugs.
- Having sex only with a partner who is **not** HIV-infected and who only has sex with you, does not shoot drugs and does not share needles and syringes.
- Using condoms and a spermicide or latex gloves (for masturbation, etc.) whenever you are unsure about your partner's infection. You can only be sure your partner is not infected through testing. You should not rely on your partner to protect your health. **You must take responsibility for yourself.**
- Not allowing another persons's blood (including menstral blood), semen, urine, or vaginal secretions to enter into your vagina, anus or mouth.
- If you are HIV-infected or think you may be, never allow your blood and other body fluids to enter into another person's body. (Always use protection.)

About Pregnancy

You should not worry about how AIDS will affect your pregnancy if you and your partner are not infected with the HIV. If you are unsure about infection, both you and your partner should consider taking the HIV anti-body test.

Women who are infected should avoid becoming pregnant because they can pass the HIV to their babies during pregnancy or at birth. Roughly 50 percent of the time, infected mothers pass the virus to their babies. Most children with AIDS become infected this way. Much less frequently, the HIV may also be passed from mother to child through the breast milk of the infected mother. Babies born infected usually become sick and die before the age of three.

Because being pregnant weakens the body's immune system, pregnancy may increase the chances that a woman infected with HIV will develop AIDS.

Get HIV/AIDS Counseling Before Getting Pregnant If:

- If you or your partner have had any risky behavior since 1977.
- If you are concerned that you or your partner may be infected.

If You Are Pregnant and Suspect HIV Infection

If you or your partner may be infected with the HIV (the AIDS virus), talk to your doctor or health care worker.

Artificial Insemination

Even if you are considering artificial insemination, ask the medical center representative if the donor has been tested for the HIV, or ask the semen donor.

Cesarean Birth

Some women need blood transfusions after having a cesarean birth, or for other surgery. Though infection with the HIV from donated blood is now rare, you, along with your doctor, may consider storing your blood (autologus donation) if you need a transfusion for scheduled surgery.

Table 6. Female adult/adolescent AIDS cases by exposure category, and race/ethnicity, reported through April 1990, United States

Female exposure category	White, not Hispanic No.	(%)	Black, not Hispanic No.	(%)	Hispanic No.	(%)	Asian/Pacific Islander No.	(%)	American Indian/ Alaskan Native No.	(%)	Total[4] No.	(%)
IV drug use	1,349	(41)	3,646	(57)	1,278	(52)	11	(17)	15	(56)	6,312	(52)
Hemophilia/coagulation disorder	23	(1)	4	(0)	1	(0)	—		—		28	(0)
Heterosexual contact:	919	(28)	2,006	(32)	889	(36)	25	(38)	7	(26)	3,854	(31)
Sex with IV drug user	480		1,168		747		11		3		2,415	
Sex with bisexual male	210		126		48		6		1		392	
Sex with person with hemophilia	48		5		1		1		—		55	
Born in Pattern-II country	1		482		3		1		—		488	
Sex with person born in Pattern-II country	3		34		1		—		—		38	
Sex with transfusion recipient with HIV infection	51		8		9		1		—		69	
Sex with HIV-infected person, risk not specified	126		183		80		5		3		397	
Receipt of blood transfusion, blood components, or tissue	787	(24)	241	(4)	140	(6)	23	(35)	2	(7)	1,194	(10)
Other/undetermined	234	(7)	460	(7)	136	(6)	7	(11)	3	(11)	848	(7)
Female Total	**3,312**	**(100)**	**6,357**	**(100)**	**2,444**	**(100)**	**66**	**(100)**	**27**	**(100)**	**12,236**	**(100)**

[1] Countries with a distinctive pattern of transmission termed "Pattern II" by the World Health Organization.

[2] Includes 8 transfusion recipients who received blood screened by HIV antibody, and 1 tissue recipient.

[3] "Other" refers to 2 health-care workers who seraconverted to HIV and developed AIDS after occupational exposure to HIV-infected blood "Undetermined" refers to patients whose mode of exposure to HIV is unknown. This includes patients under investigation; patients who died, were lost to follow-up or refused interview; and patients whose mode of exposure to HIV remains undetermined after investigation.

[4] Includes 2286 males and 30 females whose race ethnicity is unknown.

SOURCE: HIV/AIDS Surveillance U.S. Department of Health and Human Services, 1990.

9/Children and AIDS: What Should Parents Do?

How Children Get AIDS

It is predicted that within a few years, thousands of infants and children (under age 13) will be infected with the HIV. Many of them will develop AIDS.

Facts on Children and HIV/AIDS.

- Most children with HIV/AIDS are under age thirteen and were born of HIV-infected mothers, who passed it to them during pregnancy. The majority of HIV-infected babies become sick and die before the age of three. Most of the mothers were IV drug users or the sexual partner of men participating in high-risk behavior.
- Shortly after birth, HIV infection may also be passed to the baby through the breast milk of the infected mother. This is very rare: world-wide fewer than 10 cases have been reported.
- HIV-infected blood transfusions and blood products caused HIV infection for some children. Blood screening has now reduced the risk of infection through blood transfusions and hemophilia treatments. (See "The Safety of the Blood Supply.")
- There **have not** been any cases of young children getting AIDS from playing with other HIV-infected children.
- Children can also become infected through sexual abuse. If you know of any such cases, contact: The National Child Abuse Hot Line (toll free) 1-800-422-4453.

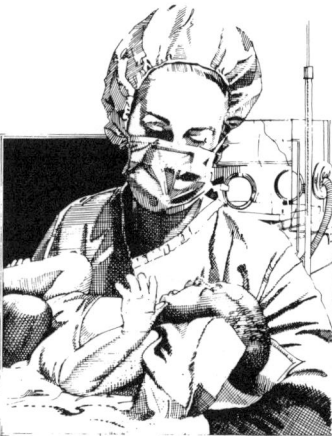

Protecting Your Children from AIDS

Talking about HIV/AIDS may seem awkward, because teaching your child about HIV infection and AIDS means talking about drugs and sex.

Discussing HIV/AIDS with Young Children

Consider these suggestions:

- Instead of waiting for your child to ask questions, **you** should begin the discussion.
- An example of a good time to start a discussion would be after viewing an AIDS-related program on television, or after reading a magazine or newspaper article on the subject.
- Listen to what your child's questions and concerns are, as well as what he or she has heard about AIDS, correcting any misinformation as you go.
- Most young children have heard about AIDS and know that it is very serious. They may be afraid. To combat this fear, they need to know basics such as:

They will not get the AIDS virus (HIV) from:
- Toilet seats.
- Swimming pools.
- Playground equipment.
- Everyday activities.
- Playing with a child whose mother or father has HIV/AIDS.
- Sitting next to a student who has HIV/AIDS.
- A teacher who has HIV/AIDS.

- Explain the facts plainly, in words that are easy for your child to understand.
- Teach your children not to pick up hypodermic needles and syringes that may be found outside or laying around.
- If your child babysits a child with AIDS, then special instructions from the infected child's family are needed.
- You and your child can find the answers together. You may want to call your local American Red Cross, an AIDS hot line, or visit your public library for more information.
- See "Information, Counseling and Support" for more points of contact.

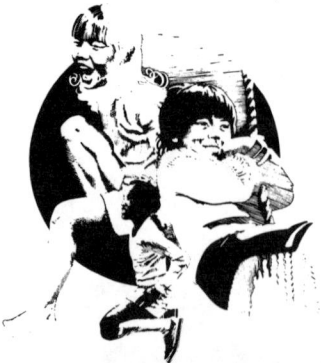

Be Aware:

Don't let fear stop your efforts to teach your children something that could save their lives.

Table 7.   Pediatric AIDS cases by exposure category, and sex, reported May 1988 through April 1989, May 1989 through April 1990; and cumulative totals, by exposure category, through April 1990, United States

Pediatric (< 13 years old) exposure category	Males May 1988-Apr. 1989 No.	(%)	Males May 1989-Apr. 1990 No.	(%)	Females May 1988-Apr. 1989 No.	(%)	Females May 1989-Apr. 1990 No.	(%)	Totals May 1988-Apr. 1989 No.	(%)	Totals May 1989-Apr. 1990 No.	(%)	Cumulative total[1] No.	(%)
Hemophilia/coagulation disorder	32	(10)	28	(8)	1	(0)	—		33	(6)	28	(4)	114	(5)
Mother with/at risk for HIV infection:	244	(76)	305	(82)	250	(91)	292	(92)	494	(83)	597	(87)	1,853	(83)
IV drug use	*128*		*148*		*119*		*132*		*247*		*280*			
Sex with IV drug user	*945*		*51*		*78*		*49*		*68*		*100*		*395*	
Sex with bisexual male	*7*		*4*		*5*		*7*		*12*		*11*		*42*	
Sex with person with hemophilia	*—*		*—*		*1*		*—*		*1*		*—*		*7*	
Born in Pattern-II country	*25*		*26*		*24*		*22*		*49*		*48*		*191*	
Sex with person born in Pattern-II country	*1*		*—*		*—*		*3*		*1*		*3*		*7*	
Sex with transfusion recipient with HIV infection	*2*		*1*		*3*		*3*		*5*		*4*		*10*	
Sex with HIV-infected person, risk not specified	*9*		*14*		*13*		*14*		*22*		*28*		*75*	
Receipt of blood transfusion, blood components or tissue	*1*		*6*		*8*		*6*		*9*		*12*		*38*	
Has HIV infection, risk not specified	*20*		*28*		*28*		*37*		*48*		*65*		*153*	
Receipt of blood transfusion, blood components, or tissue	36	(11)	27	(7)	16	(6)	13	(4)	52	(9)	40	(6)	226	(10)
Undetermined	8	(3)	11	(3)	8	(3)	14	(4)	16	(3)	25	(4)	55	(2)
Pediatric Total	**320**	**(100)**	**371**	**(100)**	**275**	**(100)**	**319**	**(100)**	**595**	**(100)**	**690**	**(100)**	**2,258**	**(100)**

[1] Includes 3 patients known to be infected with human immunodeficiency virus type 2 (HIV-2). See MMWR 1989, 38 572-580

[2] Countries with distinctive pattern of transmission termed patient II by the World Health Organization.

[3] Includes 8 transfusion recipients who received blood screened by HIV antibody, and 1 tissue recipient.

[4] "Other" refers to 2 health-care workers who seroconvened to HIV and developed AIDS after occupational exposure to HIV-infected blood. "Undetermined" refers to patients whose mode of exposure to HIV is unknown. This includes patients under investigation, patients who died, were lost to follow-up or refused interview, and patients whose mode of exposure to HIV remains undetermined after investigation.

SOURCE: HIV/AIDS Surveillance U.S. Department of Health and Human Services, 1990.

10/Teenagers and AIDS

Why Should Teens Know About AIDS?

Teens should know about HIV infection and AIDS because they often take risks with sex, drugs and alcohol.

Studies show that two-thirds of all teens have had sex before the age of 18. They don't think they are at risk, or that AIDS can happen to them. Each year, one out of seven teens gets a sexually transmitted disease. And one out of ten teenage girls gets pregnant.

Furthermore, studies show that one out of five people with AIDS today are age 20 to 30. Since it takes 10 years or longer for symptoms to appear, these people may have become infected while still in their teens.

What Can Parents Do?

Parents should know the facts about HIV/AIDS and discuss them with their children. They can help their children learn how the HIV (the AIDS virus) is spread, and how it is not spread.

Though AIDS is a frightening disease, we can't let our fear stop us from protecting our children. It's up to us to teach them the facts.

To assist in preventing the spread of the AIDS virus among young people, parents and children need to talk about sex and drugs.

Discussions concerning sex and drugs with your children also give you the opportunity to share family values. AIDS prevention is most effective when young people hear the message early. Teens need to know the truth about HIV infection and AIDS.

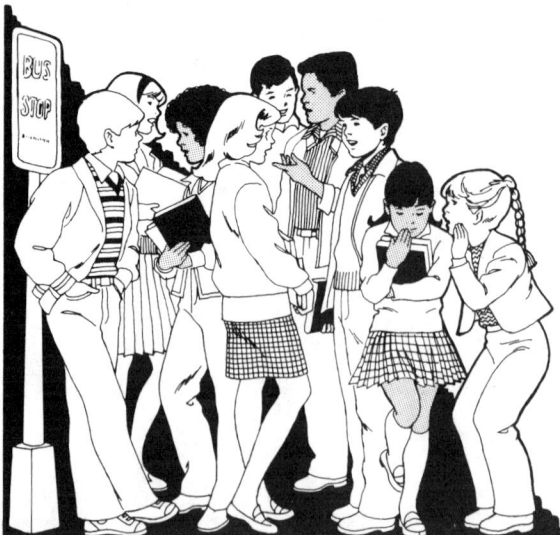

What Else Can Parents Do?

- As a parent you can play a significant role in the AIDS education and awareness process. Learn the facts and share information about the HIV and AIDS with your teens.
- If the subject of AIDS comes up, talk openly about it. And if it doesn't come up, don't wait. Teens need to know.
- Local schools have a responsibility to ensure that their students know the facts about AIDS. Find out what your child's school is doing about AIDS awareness and education. (For more information concerning teachers, schools, and school officials see "AIDS and Your Job.")

Discussing AIDS with Teens and Preteens

It's not unusual to feel uncomfortable discussing sex and drugs with teens and pre-teens. Letting them in on your feelings of discomfort may help break the ice.

When talking with your teens or pre-teens consider these suggestions:

- Completely and honestly answer all your children's questions.
- After a discussion, allow them time to think about what you have said. Don't make them feel pressured to talk.
- Let them know you are concerned about their health and care about their future.
- Recognize that being accepted by friends is very important to teens and pre-teens, especially as they get older. They may even take risks to be liked or considered popular.
- Get to know your teen's friends so you can understand what pressures they may be under.
- If your child babysits a child with HIV/AIDS, then special instructions from the infected child's family are needed.
- Make sure your child is aware of the facts about the HIV. Discuss what he or she may have learned in school, and add anything you think has been left out.
- Children can learn from their parents or a trusted older person. Also, a special class or seminar on topics like "good decision making" and "resisting peer pressure" may be helpful.

Other Essential Facts to Share with Teens and Pre-Teens

- Teens may not be clear on who may be infected with the HIV. Stress to them that the people who have died from AIDS in the United States have been: babies; male and female; rich and poor; young and old, lesbian, gay, straight, and bisexual; Caucasian, African American, Hispanic, Asian, American Indian, and Alaska Native.
- The HIV has no respect for who you are, how old you are, what your sexual orientation is, or where you live. AIDS is a deadly disease.
- Once AIDS develops, there is no chance of complete recovery, because right now there is no vaccine or cure. First and foremost, it must be prevented.
- The best protection against HIV infection is not having sex and not experimenting with drugs.
- Avoiding sex before marriage or a long-term love relationship, where both uninfected partners are faithful (sex only with that one person) is the next best protection, after abstinence, against the sexual spread of HIV infection—as long as other risky behaviors have not occured.
- One of the ways HIV infection is spread is through sex with an HIV-infected person. This includes all types of sex. The virus is passed in blood, vaginal secretions, semen and other body fluids.
- Other STDs make it easier for HIV to enter into the bloodstream. (See AIDS and Other Sexually Transmitted Diseases.")
- HIV infection is also spread through drug use by sharing used needles and syringes with an HIV-infected person. A person can get the AIDS virus from sharing even one needle and syringe with someone who is infected.
- If one of the partners has used IV drugs in the past few years or is currently sharing needles, he or she could cause HIV infection through sex. (See chapter on "Prevention.")
- Latex condoms and spermicidal foams can help prevent HIV infection if both are used properly each and every time intercourse takes place.
- The more sex partners, you have, the greater your chances of becoming infected.
- A person can get the AIDS virus from even one sexual act with an infected partner.
- Drugs and alcohol affect the judgment of both teens and adults. People are more likely to take dangerous risks and avoid protecting themselves from the HIV when they are high on drugs and/or alcohol.

- Teens and children can also become infected through sexual abuse. If you know of any such cases, contact: The National Child Abuse Hotline (toll free) 1-800-422-4453.
- Needles used for tattooing should not be used on more than one person. Tattoo artists may not take the time to clean the needles between uses.
- You can't tell if someone is infected with the AIDS virus by the way he or she looks. In order to really know if a person is HIV-infected, he or she has to be tested.
- Birth control pills and diaphragms do not protect either partner against the AIDS virus or other sexually transmitted diseases.
- AIDS can only be prevented by avoiding high-risk behaviors that spread the virus. (See "Prevention.")
- The HIV is spread through infected blood, not through casual contact that may occur at schools or other public places.

Some examples of casual contact are:
- A cough or sneeze
- A hug or handshake
- Tears or sweat
- Pets
- Eating food prepared or served by someone infected with the AIDS virus
- Toilet or shower facilities
- Swimming pools
- Spoons, forks, knives and cups
- Computers, chairs, desks or bus seats
- Drinking fountains
- Phones
- Sports equipment, etc.

Teaching Teenagers About Condoms

Prepare your children before they become sexually active. When talking to teenagers about condoms, make sure they understand the following messages:
- Condoms help prevent the spread of the HIV, the virus that causes AIDS.
- There are other benefits to using condoms. They can prevent other sexually transmitted diseases like syphilis, gonnorhea, chlamydia and genital herpes, as well as pregnancy.
- Although latex condoms with a spermicide are the best protection devices we have today, they are still not foolproof. The latex condom must be used properly with a spermicide each time to get the best protection. (See "Prevention.")
- Condoms do not completely eliminate the risk of infection with the

AIDS virus, because they may slip off, tear or break. (See "Why Condoms Fail.")

- Latex condoms can be used for all types of sex, including vaginal, oral and anal intercourse.

If Teens Are Not Sexually Active

- If a teen is not having sex or doesn't "mess around" with drugs and alcohol, **congratulations are in order!** These teens should be commended. They don't have to worry about getting HIV/AIDS.

If Teens Are Sexually Active

- Each partner should take responsibility for his or her own protection.
- Boys should use a condom each time.
- Girls should make their boyfriends use a latex condom with a spermicide. Caution: **Never use a spermicide without a condom.**
- Sexually active teens (both girls and boys) should keep condoms handy.
- Don't think it can't happen to your child. It can.
- Take the proper precautions now!

Be Aware:

There are specific guidelines for condom use outlined under "Prevention," in the section called "How to Use a Condom Effectively."

- Condoms must be used correctly.
- Condoms must be used each time sexual intercourse occurs.
- Condoms must be used with a spermicide to further reduce risk.
- Both products must be stored properly.

Table 8. **AIDS cases in Adolescents (13-19 years old) and Adults under age 25,** by exposure category, reported May 1988 through April 1989, May 1989 through April 1990, and cumulative totals through April 1990, United States.

Exposure category	13-19 years old						20-24 years old					
	May 1988-Apr. 1989		May 1989-Apr. 1990		Cumulative total		May 1988-Apr. 1989		May 1989-Apr. 1990		Cumulative total	
	No.	(%)	No.	(%)	No.	(%)	No.	(%)	No.	(%)	No.	(%)
Male homosexual/bisexual contact	32	(28)	33	(24)	145	(28)	819	(57)	802	(51)	3,254	(57)
Intravenous (IV) drug use (female and heterosexual male)	17	(15)	15	(11)	59	(12)	236	(16)	292	(19)	903	(16)
Male homosexual/bisexual contact and IV drug use	5	(4)	3	(2)	23	(4)	116	(8)	135	(9)	534	(9)
Hemophilia/coagulation disorder	34	(30)	39	(28)	157	(31)	41	(3)	37	(2)	148	(3)
Heterosexual contact:	13	(11)	25	(18)	62	(12)	137	(10)	175	(11)	503	(9)
Sex with IV drug user	*7*		*17*		*37*		*87*		*96*		*271*	
Sex with bisexual male	*—*		*1*		*3*		*12*		*6*		*43*	
Sex with person with hemophilia	*—*		*1*		*1*		*4*		*7*		*14*	
Born in Pattern-II[1] country	*3*		*2*		*13*		*12*		*26*		*100*	
Sex with person born in Pattern-II country	*—*		*—*		*—*		*—*		*4*		*6*	
Sex with transfusion recipient with HIV infection	*—*		*—*		*—*		*—*		*3*		*4*	
Sex with HIV-infected person, risk not specified	*3*		*4*		*8*		*22*		*33*		*65*	
Receipt of blood transfusion, blood components, or tissue	14	(12)	3	(2)	38	(7)	25	(2)	13	(1)	86	(2)
Undetermined[2]	—		19	(14)	29	(6)	57	(4)	106	(7)	242	(4)
Adolescent Total	**115**	**(100)**	**137**	**(100)**	**513**	**(100)**	**1,431**	**(100)**	**1,560**	**(100)**	**5,670**	**(100)**

[1] Countries with a distinctive pattern of transmission termed ''Pattern II'' by the World Health Organization.

[2] ''Undetermined'' refers to patients whose mode of exposure to HIV is unknown. This includes patients under investigation; patients who died, were lost to follow-up, or refused interview; and patients whose mode of exposure to HIV remains undetermined after investigation. See Figure 4.

SOURCE: HIV/AIDS Surveillance U.S. Department of Health and Human Services, May 1990.

11/AIDS and Other Sexually Transmitted Diseases

The Connection

Clinicians and scientists are finding that the presence of other sexually transmitted diseases serves as an indicator of three things:

1. More People are Vulnerable to HIV Infection

Studies in the U.S. and in Africa have shown that genital sores, warts, etc., facilitate the entry of the HIV into the bloodstream by increasing the exposure to blood. A rise in sexually transmitted diseases (STDs) means that a greater number of people are now vulnerable to HIV infection.

2. The Presence of Other STDs Complicates Treatment of HIV/AIDS

The incidence of genital warts and other diseases signals a suppressed immune system. Treating syphilis cases can be complicated by HIV infection, and vice versa. Because the presence of a sexually transmitted disease signals unsafe sexual practices, some doctors are recommending that a person be tested for HIV infection each time a STD is diagnosed.

3. AIDS Education Can Help with Other STDs as Well

If AIDS education programs are successful, then they will also assist in the reduction of other sexually transmitted diseases such as syphilis, gonorrhea and herpes.

12/Living With AIDS: Two HIV-Infected People Share Their Experience

1. Terri

Seemingly normal, Terri is an attractive 33-year-old African American female, who contracted the AIDS virus from her late husband, possibly as long as eight years ago. Doctors aren't sure, because it was eight years after her husband developed symptoms that he was properly diagnosed with AIDS. Terri currently has no symptoms of the virus. Unfortunately, she passed the infection on to her two-year-old daughter, who has AIDS and cerebral palsy. Terri's life isn't easy, but she's coping. She recently moved from her parents home, where she lived after her husband's death, into a nearby two-bedroom apartment.

What follows is part of an interview with Terri. As the evening sun came through her living room window, Terri talked about how HIV/AIDS has affected her life.

Q: Why did you decide to do this interview?

A: Because I think it's good for people to know as much as they can. It's good for them, in terms of protecting themselves and knowing what's of real danger and risk and what isn't. And it's good for those of us who are infected. We don't have to worry about them being concerned about being around us or around our children. It benefits both ends. I try to do what I can to make that happen.

Q: You were pregnant when you discovered you and your husband were HIV-positive. Did that present a greater problem?

A: At that point the doctor I went to didn't know a whole lot about what that (being HIV-positive) meant and what the chances were (that my baby would be born with AIDS). The information that he gave me wasn't what we know now in terms of the possibility of transmission. So he told me to go ahead and have the baby.

Q: How many months pregnant were you?

A: I was only about six to eight weeks pregnant when I found out, so there was the opportunity to terminate the pregnancy. At that time my doctor said that there was about a 75 percent chance that she (my daughter) would be O.K. But we (my husband and I) had tried for a couple of years and had prayed about it very hard and very diligently so we decided that we would take that risk.

Q: How did your husband get the virus?

A: From what we know, he had experimented with drugs in 1977. He and his brother had shared needles. His brother had been in the military in Vietnam and had come back. They had been experimenting with drugs. I would think that is how it was transmitted from his brother to to him.

Q: How did you feel when you found out? Were you angry?

A: Well, not when I found out. I wasn't mad—I was terrified. I was thinking mostly of my child and what we were going to do about that situation. We were married—had been for eight years. We were living away from home and neither of us had family there. We just had each other. I know that if he had any idea of what he was doing at the time, he would have taken precautions. It wasn't his fault that it happened. There were times when I got angry, and those times were when my daughter was very very sick. Then I felt anger. But when I found out, it was a matter of how we were going to make it through this.

Q: When your daughter was sick, did you ever seek the help of support groups?

A: There (in the city where we lived), we did not. We chose to be very secretive about it. Our parents did not know until after she was about six months old. We had talked with her doctor and we were living away from our parents and there was not much contact. And we felt that we just wanted to deal with it by ourselves. So we chose to do that as long as we could.

Q: When your parents found out were they very supportive?

A: My parents were very concerned about me and my daughter. As things got worse they tried to support us as best they could. They really wanted my daughter and me to come home. There was some problem with the relationship between my mother and my husband because of it. Eventually, as my husband's condition worsened, I had to ask his parents to take him for a while. They supported us as best they could, but they had problems with it too. And not so much afraid of becoming infected, but what it meant to the whole family.

Q: What did this mean to your family?

A: They feared what other people might think. They felt that I had married him and should stay with him until death do we part. And of course, that is what we would have preferred happen. But it got to the point where my daughter came down with pneumocystis in December 86 and she was in the hospital for six weeks. She came out in late January and he went in in March and was there for about 10 days. He came out and then (later on) went back in April, May and June. While he was in, she went in late May and June. Then she came out, and he came out. They were in two different hospitals—she was in a children's hospital on a separate end of town and I was working, trying to see the two of them.

Q: How did you do it?

A: Well, I did it as long as I could, and when I couldn't do anymore I told them (our families) I was selling the house and that I had to get my daughter here to Duke (Duke University Medical Center). She's on a protocol that they didn't have in the city where I was. My husband and I talked about it and decided that this was what we needed to do. He could not work, so his family eventually had to take him.

Q: What kind of treatment is your daughter on?

A: She takes AZT four times a day.

Q: Are you taking the medication also?

A: I'm on a protocol also. I believe I'm on AZT but it's an experimental protocol. Some people get a small dose. Some people get a high dose and some people get no dose at all. I don't know exactly what I'm taking. It may be sugar for all I know.

Q: Do you think it's helping? You look great.

A: Well, I've not had any symptoms. My immune system is not totally normal. My counts are down, but they're not dangerously down. And, I've had no symptoms.

Q: You said earlier that you've had the virus for eight years. Most people develop symptoms earlier than that, don't they?

A: A lot of people think you get AIDS right away. Though I don't know exactly when I became infected, most likely it was early on in the marriage I would imagine, rather than later. But, there is no way to really tell.

Q: There really are a lot of misconceptions about AIDS. What are some of the ones you're familiar with?

A: People think we (people with AIDS) are drug addicts, gay people, black and dirty. I think that they think they're all going die almost immediately and that there is no hope. And I think that some people don't want to read and understand how the virus is transmitted.

Q: What do you see in your daughter's future?

A: That's probably one of the touchiest and the most difficult things I have to deal with. I don't know. Especially since some of the children (with AIDS) are quite normal other than being infected. If it weren't for that and her motor skills, I would say it would be as normal as mine, except that she'd probably be sick a lot more than the normal person.

Q: Is she like any other child with cerebral palsy?

A: Yes. It's difficult because when you have a child, you expect to have a baby for maybe a year but even within that time they eventually hold a bottle, move around, and find ways to entertain themselves, so you don't have an infant for any more than six months. My daughter can't hold a bottle, she can't sit up, and probably worst of all, she can't talk. So, it's hard to communicate and to know what she wants and know what she feels and how she feels about the way she is. That bothers me. I wish we could at least talk to each other. But she's in therapy and we're trying to figure out a way she can communicate with her eyes.

Q: What about your future?

A: I don't know. I don't look too far into the future. Not because I'm afraid of it, but because it's easier just to go day by day. I thought I'd probably live my life alone—me and my daughter—but surprisingly, that may not have to be so. There are people who are bright enough to love you and accept you for what you are. And to accept me is to accept that I'm HIV-positive and what that could mean for them.

Q: What about intimacy?

A: Sex is certainly different. There's no casual sex and it's very hard in terms of a relationship, to take the risk to develop one, because very early on you have to let a person know that you're HIV-positive. You may not have to do it on the first date but sometime within a couple of weeks, there's going to be a time when you can't put a person off any longer. You'll just have to say it and at that point you really leave yourself open to whatever. You have to be really careful about the people you choose because you don't want to get blasted out or rejected. Nobody wants to be rejected. I was fortunate in that the person I met, took the time to get to know me as a friend. Now I know that what I thought would never be, is possible.

Q: If you could be or do anything in the world that you wanted, what would it be?

A: I'd get rid of this virus. I'd like my husband back. I'd like my daughter well. I guess that's it.

2. Charles

Carefully applied opaque make-up barely conceals the dark *Kaposi's Sarcoma* lesions that cover Charles' face. Once the expressive face of an actor, it is now swollen with dark blotches. He is a six-foot-four Caucasian male, weighing about 150 pounds. Charles is 35 years old. He often wears his shirt collars high to hide the visual signs of a disease that so many don't understand.

Charles found out that he had AIDS in December 1987, right before Christmas. He went to the doctor when he discovered six dark blotches on his body. After a biopsy at a major medical center, doctors told Charles he had AIDS. The following is an excerpt of a conversation with Charles one summer afternoon, in his studio apartment. He talked of his quest to educate people about AIDS and how he's coping with the disease.

It's Charles' mission to help people understand. He frequently gives talks to enlighten the public, especially teenagers, on the facts about AIDS. "People need to know that statistically, people in the 20 to 30 year-old age groups were infected with the virus as many as ten years ago. Some of these folks indeed may have been infected with the virus when they were teenagers. We need to bring to light that teenagers do have sex, so—they need to have safe sex, if any at all."

Q: Why do you speak to the public about AIDS as much as you do?

A: It's very fulfilling. It's a very strengthening experience. It's sort of funny, when I get to the end of a talk, people are very thankful for my being there—I always let them know that I'm kind of in a selfish situation. I get a great deal out of going out and talking about what it's like to be alive with AIDS—some of the things that I've lived through and some of the things friends of mine have experienced—because I feel like education is indeed the key. Hatred and bigotry are not going to be dispelled without people willing to sit down and talk about what's going on.

Q: In your talks with people, what impression do you get that they are really accepting of the fact that AIDS can happen to them?

A: I think many people are having problems looking past their fear to the realistic fact that most people with AIDS are not a threat to mainstream society. There's a radical decrease in the gay population, for example, of the incidence of new cases of the disease. This says to me that the message to that population, for the most part, has gotten out. Currently, AIDS is on the rise in the heterosexual community and that's really sad, because there's no need for other people to contract this disease any longer.

Q: What can we do? What's really going to be the thing that's going to hit home?

A: It's really a hard and sad lesson because many people are not going to listen until AIDS actually touches their lives and by that, I mean someone that they've known from high school dies of AIDS, someone that they've dated in the past contracts the disease. Many people are still saying, "it's not going to get me" and that's an O.K. attitude to have, provided you couple that with responsible attitudes, practices and behaviors.

Q: Do you think everyone should be tested?

A: I could go along with not being tested (if you're in a high risk group) as long as you've made behavioral changes in your life. It's not real important whether you're HIV-positive or negative, provided you're behaving responsibly.

Q: What was your reaction when you found out you had AIDS?

A: I knew enough about AIDS and enough about my own sexual history to not really be too terribly taken aback by that news. I mean emotionally yes, there was a lot of stuff to deal with, but I wasn't radically shocked. I've been a rather promiscuous person in the past, so discovering that I had AIDS was not real shocking news like it might be to someone who has only had sex a couple of times. I'd had lots and lots of contacts, many of which were anonymous.

Q: Even when you were promiscuous, as you say, you knew the potential was there. Didn't you care?

A: I didn't really know the potential for AIDS was there until the early 80's. It was at that point in time that I changed my behavior. I began safe sex practices. But prior to that point in time I didn't. I "came out" when I was 17 and became publicly known as a gay person, and had been having sex since I was 13 years old—that's 22 years. I'm currently 35. I suspect I was infected with the virus prior to the time we really realized that here was a disease that was not just your standard STD that could be cured with penicillin or a variety of antibiotics. But when the news came out about AIDS transmission methods, I did change my behavioral practices.

Q: How did you feel?

A: I was shocked, hurt. Emotionally, kind of devastated. I found out right around Christmas. My anxiety level went right through the ceiling. You know, AIDS doesn't get a lot of good press.

Q: What kind of treatment are you on?

A: I was on AZT for about the first year and three months and I also underwent chemotherapy for over a year. I recently have changed my course of pursuit and am looking more toward eastern medicine and alternative healing techniques. When I stopped doing chemotherapy, I had reached a point where I was extremely tired all the time—very little energy to do anything. Cooking and cleaning up my dishes was the most I could muster in a day's time. And even that was a challenge. Two weeks after I stopped chemotherapy I had this radical amount of energy. So I felt like the chemotherapy was making me sick. And it's sort of like deciding where the balance is for you. It's a very personal decision. For me I had to weigh out—do I want longer survival with no quality in the hope that something will come up between now and whenever, or do I want my quality and possibly sacrifice a little bit of time? My feeling is that I can have both. I've started working with an acupuncture therapist and with a person who teaches an oriental method of channeling energy into the body and both those things, I think, are working.

Q: Did you tell your family immediately once you found out?

A: No, not right away. I found out in December 1987 at that point in time I also found out I was coming down with *Pneumocystis Pneumonia* and the first three weeks in January, I spent flat on my back, very, very ill physically and very depleted mentally. I was not in any way able to tell my family. I didn't have the physical or emotional strength that I knew it would require to tell them. So they didn't find out 'til the end of January. My mother yelled at me for not telling her sooner.

Q: What kind of support have you recieved from them?

A: It's sort of strange the way that they've been supportive. They found out that I had AIDS in January of 1988 and they didn't come to visit me until January 1989. So it was an entire year before they started to come visit and that was because at Christmas last year, I got very verbal about their waiting so long. I expressed my concern to my Mom in particular that after I'm dead, it's too late to visit then.

Q: What would you tell parents of persons with AIDS?

A: Parents need to be emotionally supportive of someone who's dealing with this disease. They need to listen very carefully and just be there. That's the most important thing. Be there in a nonjudgmental, non-critical, supportive kind of way. AIDS is not a gay disease. Granted it did start in that population, but the reason it spread as far as it did was the lack of education and funding. Because it did start with gay males, society wanted to sort of turn its head away. And that's sort of sad that we've reached a period in society where people are expendable.

Q: Were you employed?

A: Yes I was. I continued to work through March 1988. In which time, I began to see the company taking privileges away from me. I was a supervisor and had people working for me. I came in one morning and started to log onto the payroll system to look at the hours of my employees and to scan over what was in the computer and I couldn't get on the system. I was shocked and went to the fellow who was in control of the system and he just told me to talk to my supervisor, which seemed pretty cold at that point in time.

Q: How did you feel about the way your dismissal was handled?

A: Later reflecting on it, there wasn't a whole lot he could say; he had been given his instructions. But about that same time, I heard rumors that they were going to fire me, so I took a medical disability. I also was growing physically more and more tired. I can't help but feel that it had been affecting my job performance somewhat. But I feel like a more appropriate procedure could have been taken. Technically, the procedures that were on the books with this company would have been to call me down and talk with me about my job performance, set some goals.

Q: How should companies set AIDS policy?

A: People with AIDS or who are HIV-positive are quite capable physi-cally of carrying out their duties. They should be permitted to remain employed, provided they can still do their work. If job performance is indeed slipping and they are not able to do the work done previously, moving them around within the company might be a possiblity, or sug-gesting that they retire or whatever. But I think the most important part is communication. It should be a two-way street, not a one-way power play, because I think people who have this disease do realize they have some limitations.

Q: You don't delude yourself at all about this disease. How do you accept it?

A: I can't change where I'm at. I feel like the best thing for me to do is to continue living with AIDS. I'm pretty logical, a fairly deep thinker, able to look at situations, take two steps back from the frame and be able to see the big picture. I don't become so totally immersed in the forest that I can't see the trees.

Q: What does your future hold?

A: I sort of take one day at a time. I do have goals, I've not given up all my dreams and aspirations. Initially, yes there was a tendency to let go of all my dreams, but I came to the conclusion that I'm still alive, right up to the time they put me in the box. And I'm not going to let go of my dreams. I think it's important to continue to strive to do the things that you can and to not buy too far into the media's "everybody dies" kind of attitude. If you really look at that on a base level, everybody dies, yes indeed, no matter who you are, no matter where you're at, eventually everyone dies . . . we just don't know when. So, you strive to live your life as positively as you can.

Charles died in September of 1990.

Appendices:
13/AIDS Info., Counseling and Support

Find help in your own state—Departments of Health

Alabama
(205) 284-3553

Alaska
(907) 561-4406

Arizona
(602) 230-5843

Arkansas
(501) 661-2395

California
(916) 445-0553

Colorado
(303) 331-8320

Connecticut
(203) 566-4492

Delaware
(302) 995-8422

District of Columbia
(202) 332-AIDS

Florida
(904) 488-2905

Georgia
(404) 730-1401

Hawaii
(808) 922-1313

Idaho
(208) 334-5937

Illinois
(312) 744-8500

Indiana
(317) 456-2408

Iowa
(515) 281-5424

West Virginia
(304) 348-5358

Kansas
(913) 296-5641

Kentucky
(502) 564-4478

Louisiana
(504) 342-1792

Maine
(207) 289-3747

Maryland
(301) 945-AIDS

Massachusetts
(617) 727-0368

Michigan
(517) 335-8371

Minnesota
(612) 623-5414

Mississippi
(601) 960-7714

Missouri
(816) 353-9902

Montana
(800) 233-6668

Nebraska
(402) 471-2937

Nevada
(702) 385-1291

New Hampshire
(603) 271-4487

New Jersey
(609) 984-6050

New Mexico
(505) 984-0911

New York
(518) 473-0641

North Carolina
(919) 733-3419

North Dakota
(701) 224-2378

Ohio
(614) 466-4643

Oklahoma
(405) 271-4061

Oregon
(503) 229-5792

Pennsylvania
(717) 787-3350

Rhode Island
(401) 277-2320

South Carolina
(803) 734-5482

South Dakota
(605) 773-3364

Tennessee
(615) 741-7247

Texas
(512) 458-7504

Utah
(801) 538-6191

Vermont
(802) 863-7240

Virginia
(804) 786-6267

Washington
(206) 361-2914

Wisconsin
(608) 267-3583

Wyoming
(307) 777-7953

Source: U.S. Department of Health and Human Services, CDC MMWR Supplement, No. S-6

AIDS Information Hotlines, State-by-State

National AIDS Hotline: 1-800-342-AIDS
(Spanish) 1-100-244-SIDA
(TTY/TDD) 1-800-234-7889
CDC Printed Materials: 404-639-3534
CDC Recorded Information: 1-800-342-2437
Alabama: 800-455-3741
Alaska: 800-478-2437
Arizona: 800-334-1540
Arkansas: 800-445-7720
California:
• Northern California: 800-367-2437
• Southern California: 800-922-2437
Caroline Islands/Micronesia: 011-691-9-619
Colorado: 303-830-2437
Connecticut: 203-566-1157
Delaware: 302-995-8422
District of Columbia: 202-332-2437
Florida: 1-800-352-2437
Georgia: 1-800-551-2728
Guam: 011-671-0734-2947
Hawaii: 808-922-1313
• Kauai: 808-241-3495
• Maui: 808-243-5288
• Hawaii: 808- 933-4276
• Oahu: 808-735-5303
Idaho: 208-334-5944
Illinois: 1-800-243-2437
Indiana: 317-633-8406
Iowa: 800-532-3301
Kansas: 800-232-0040
Kentucky: 1-800-654-2437
Louisiana: 1-800-992-4379
Maine: 800-851-2437
Marianas Islands/Saipan: 011-670-234-8950
Marshall Islands: 011-692-9-3487
Maryland: 1-800-638-6252
Massachusetts: 800-235-2331
• Boston: 617-534-5916
Michigan: 517-335-8371
• Wellness Network, Inc. Hotline: 1-800-872-2437

Minnesota: 1-800-248-AIDS
Mississippi: 1-800-826-2961
Montana: 406-444-4740
- Billings: 406-252-1212
Nebraska: 800-782-2437
Nevada:
- Reno: 702-329-2437
- Las Vegas: 702-383-1393
New Jersey: 800-624-2377
New Mexico: 505-827-0006
New York: 800-462-1884
North Carolina: 919-733-7301
North Dakota: 800-592-1861
Ohio: 1-800-332-2437
Oklahoma:
- Oklahoma City area: 405-271-6434
- Enid area: 405-242-5555
Oregon: 503-229-5792
- Portland: 503-223-5907
Pennsylvania: 1-800-692-7254
Puerto Rico: 809-765-1010
Rhode Island:1-800-726-3010
South Carolina: 1-800-322-2437
South Dakota: 800-472-2180
Tennessee: 1-800-342-2437
Texas:
- Dallas: 214-559-2437
- Houston: 713-524-2437
Utah: 800-843-9388
Vermont: 800-882-2437
Virginia: 1-800-533-4148
Washington: 800-272-2437
West Virginia: 1-800-642-8244
Wisconsin: 1-800-334-2437
- Milwaukee area: (414) 273-2437
Wyoming: 307-777-7953

Source: San Francisco AIDS Foundation "AIDS in the Workplace, A Guide for Employees" (Data updated for accuracy)

National Help Organizations: Telephone Hotlines

National AIDS Information Hotline:
U.S. Public Health Service
Atlanta, Georgia (24 hours, daily)
1-800-342-AIDS
1-800-342-2437

The Spanish Hotline
1-800-344-7432 (SIDA)

Hotline for the Hearing Impaired
1-800-243-7889

National Sexually Transmitted
Diseases/American Social
Health Association
1-800-227-8922

AIDS Project Los Angeles
6721 Romaine St.
Los Angeles, California 90038
213-962-1600

Area-specific Toll-free Numbers:
- 1-213-876-AIDS
  (for Los Angeles only)
- 1-800-553-AIDS
  (for the Hearing Impaired)
- 1-800-222-SIDA
  (for Spanish-speaking people)

AIDS Information and Literature

U.S. Public Health Service
Public Affairs Office
Hubert H. Humphrey Bldg.
Room 725-H
200 Independence Ave., SW
Washington, DC 20201
(202) 245-6867

San Francisco AIDS Foundation
333 Valencia Street
San Francisco, CA 94103
(415) 863-2437

American Association of Physicians for Human Rights
P.O. Box 14366
San Francisco, CA 94114
(415) 558-9353

Gay Men's Health Crisis
P.O. Box 274
132 W. 24th Street
New York, NY 10011
(212) 807-6655

Hispanic AIDS Forum
c/o APRED
121 Avenue of the Americas
New York, NY 10013
(212) 966-6336

Child Help U.S.A.
P.O. Box 630
Hollywood, CA 90028
1-800-422-4453
(can give local contacts
and literature)

Local Red Cross Chapter or **American Red Cross**
AIDS Education Office
430 17th Street, NW
Washington, D.C. 20006
(202) 639-3223

Minority Task Force on AIDS
c/o New York City
Council of Churches
475 Riverside Drive, Rm. 456
New York, NY 10115
(212) 870-2120

National Coalition of Hispanic Health and Human Services (COSSMHO)
1030 15th Street, N.W./Ste 1053
Washington, D.C. 20005
1-202-387-5000

Research Organizations

American Foundation for AIDS Research
5900 Wilshire Boulevard/2nd Floor East
Los Angeles, CA 90036
1-213-857-5900

Support Groups

Shanti Foundation
6855 Santa Monica Boulevard
Suite 408
Los Angeles, California 90038
1-213-962-8197

AIDS Action Counsel
2033 M. St., NW
Suite 802
Washington, D.C. 20036
1-202-293-2886

Find Help in Your Local Area

- See your doctor.
- Call your local chapter of the American Red Cross.
- Seek out local AIDS service organizations (contact your local Red Cross for information on these organizations in your community)
- Contact your local health department.

Be Aware:

For Drug Treatment call the National Treatment Referral Hotline
1-800-662-HELP

Also, see the following chapter: "Drug Abuse and Alcoholism Treatment and Prevention Programs."

14/Drug Abuse and Alcohol Treatment and Prevention Programs

As discussed earlier in "Drug Abuse and AIDS," much of the cause for the spread of the HIV is due to the abuse of drugs and alcohol. For those who need help in stopping the substance abuse habit, what follows is a listing of facilities responsible for the provision of alcoholism and drug abuse treatment and prevention services throughout the United States.

If you need assistance with one or both of these problems, there are people out there who care and are ready and waiting to help you. There are more than 8,689 federal, state, local and private treatment and prevention programs in this country. The handbook lists two points of contact for each state.

By contacting any of the programs listed here you, can get help and/or find a program within or closer to your city.

Key

For each facility listed, there is a coding line shown. This code line will enable you to determine at a glance, the Orientation, Unit's Function, Environment or Type of Care, and Selected Special Program information at each unit. Study the codes briefly, then look for your state's entry.

Orientation

A	=	Alcoholism Services only
D	=	Drug Abuse Services only
AD	=	Both Alcoholism and Drug Services

Environment/Type of Care

I	=	Hospital/Inpatient
R	=	Residential
O	=	Out patient

Unit Function

TX	=	Treatment Unit
CI	=	Central Intake Unit
PV	=	Prevention Unit
MM	=	Methadone Maintenance
OT	=	Other Unit

Selected Special Programs:

W	=	Women
Y	=	Youth
E	=	Elderly
B	=	African Americans
H	=	Hispanics
AI	=	American Indians/ Alaska Natives
IH	=	Impaired Health Professionals
PI	=	Public Inebriates
CU	=	Cocaine Users
IV	=	IV Drug Users
DT	=	Detoxification
EA	=	EAP Program Services
DW	=	DWI/ASAP Services

Treatment Facilities and State Authorities

Listed below is one facility per state, along with a state authority for each state. In addition, there are many treatment programs throughout your state. If you cannot find the code that you are looking for under the facility listed, call the state authority listed for your state. That office will be able to refer you to the program nearest you which offers that particular treatment service which you are looking for.

Facility	State Authority

Alabama

Univ. of Alabama at Birmingham
UAB Substance Abuse Programs
3015 7th Avenue South
Birmingham AL 35233
(205) 934-2118
** AD O Y IH CU IV TX
CI MM **

Jim Laney, Director
Division Substance Abuse
   Community Programs
Department of Mental Health
200 Interstate Park Dr., Box 3710
Montgomery, AL 36193
(205) 270-4648

Alaska

Alaska Counseling
3010 Davis Road
Room B-6
Fairbanks, AK 99707
(907) 451-8160
** AD O W Y B H AI IH CU EA
DW TX CI PV OT **

Matthew Felix, Coordinator
Office of Alcoholism and Drug
   Abuse
Department of Health and
   Social Services
Pouch H-05-F
Juneau, AK 99811
(907) 586-6201

American Samoa

Facility not listed,
contact your State Authority.

Fualaau Hanipale
Assistant Director
Social Services Division
Alcohol and Drug Program
   Government of American
   Somoa
Pago Pago, A.S. 96799

Facility	State Authority

Arizona

Phoenix Camelback Hospital
Chemical Dependency Programs
5055 North 34th Street
Phoenix, AZ 85018
(602) 955-6200
** AD I Y IV TX **

Gwen Smith, Program
    Representative
    for Alcoholism
Office of Community
    Behavioral Health
Arizona Department of
    Health Services
201 E. Jefferson / Suite 400-A
Phoenix, AZ 85034

Arkansas

Family Service Agency of
    Central Arkansas
2700 North Willow Street
North Little Rock, AR 72115
(501) 758-1516
** AD O IV EA DW TX CI PV **

Paul T. Behnke, Director
Office of Alcohol and Drug
    Abuse Prevention
Donaghey Plaza, North
Suite 400
Little Rock, AR 72203-1437
(501) 682-6650

California

Alternative Action Programs
2511 South Barrington Avenue
Los Angeles, CA 90064
(213) 479-8353
** AD O W Y E H PI CU IV EA
DW TX CI PV **

Chaucey Veatch III, Director
Dept. of Alcohol and
    Drug Programs
111 Capital Mall, Suite 450
Sacremento, CA 95814
(916) 445-0834

Colorado

Centre at Porter Hospital
Substance Abuse Program
2525 South Downing Street
Denver, CO 80210
(303) 778-5774
** AD I O IV DT DW TX CI PV **

Robert Aukerman, Director
Alcohol and Drug Abuse Division
Department of Health
400 S. Colorado Blvd.
4th Floor/Suite 410
Denver, CO 80220
(303) 331-6530

Facility	State Authority

Connecticut
Community Health Services
Comprehensive Substance
  Abuse Program
520 Albany Avenue
Hartford, CT 06120
(203) 249-9625
** AD O W Y E B H IV EA DW
TX PV **

Donald J. McConell, Exec. Director
Connecticut Alcohol and Drug
    Abuse Commission
999 Asylum Avenue, 3rd Floor
Hartford, CT 06105
(203) 566-4145

Delaware
Recovery Center of Delaware
Kirkwood Detox
Kirkwood Highway
Wilmington, DE 19808
(302) 995-8610
** AD R IV DT TX PV **

Neil Meisler, Director
Deleware Division of
    Alcoholism, Drug Abuse and
    Mental Health
1901 N. Dupont Highway
Newcastle, DE 19720
(302) 421-6101

District of Columbia
Karrick Hall
Drug Treatment Center
19th and Massachusetts Ave., S.E.
Washington, DC 20003
(202) 727-5770
** AD O W H IH CU IV
TX CI PV **

Simon Holliday, Chief
Health Planning and
  Development
1875 Connecticut Avenue, NW
Washington, DC 20009
(202) 673-7481

Florida
Community Health of South
  Dade, Inc.
CMHC Substance Abuse Services
10300 SW 216th Street
Miami, FL 33190
(305) 252-4840
** AD I R O H DT EA TX CI PV **

Linda Lewis, Administrator
Alcohol and Drug Abuse
  Program Department of Health
  and Rehabilitative Services
1317 Winewood Boulevard
Tallahassee, FL 32301
(904) 488-0900

Facility	State Authority

Georgia
Dekalb Substance Abuse Services
Dekalb Addiction Clinic
1260 Briarcliff Road, NE
Atlanta, GA 30306
(404) 894-5808
** AD O W Y CU IV DW TX
CI PV **

Patricia Redmond, Director
Alcohol and Drug
  Services Section
878 Peachtree Street, NE
Suite 318
Atlanta, GA 30309
(404) 894-6352

Guam
Facility not listed,
call your State
Authority.

Joseph A. Cameron
Director
Dept. of Mental Health
  and Substance Abuse
Box 9400
Tamuning, Guam 96911
(671) 646-9262 or 9269

Hawaii
Anodyne, Inc.
DUI and Chemical Dependency
  Treatment Programs
1188 Bishop Street
Suite 3204
Honolulu, HI 96813
(808) 545-7706
** AD O W IH CU EA DW
TX OT **

Patricia Hunter
Acting Branch Chief
Alcohol and Drug
  Abuse Branch
Department of Health
Honolulu, HI 96801
(808) 586-4007

Idaho
Health Services Corporation
DBA New Hope Center
141 Warm Springs Avenue
Boise, ID 83712
(208) 336-5454
** AD I O IV DT EA DW
TX CI PV OT **

Ray Winterowd, Chief
Bureau of Substance Abuse
  and Social Services
Department of Health
  and Welfare
450 W. State Street / 7th Floor
Boise, ID 83720
(208) 334-5935

Facility	State Authority

Illinois
Brotherhood Against Slavery
  to Addiction
Drug Abuse Program
3054-56 W. Cermak Road
Chicago, IL 60623
(312) 521-7007
**** D O B H CU IV DT TX
CI MM ****

William T. Atkins, Director
Illinois Department of Alcoholism
  and Substance Abuse
100 W. Randolph Street
Suite 5-600
Chicago, IL 60601
(312) 814-3840

Indiana
SW Indiana Mental Health Center,
  Inc.
Substance Abuse Services
613 Cherry Street
Evansville, IN 47713
(812) 423-7791, Ext. 293
** Y E IV EA DW TX CI PV **

Joseph E. Mills, Director
Division of Addiction Services
Department of Mental Health
117 East Washington Street
Indianapolis, IN 46204
(317) 232-7816

Iowa
Intersectional United Advanced
  Planning Center (IUAP)
2323 Forest Avenue
Des Moines, IA 50311
(515) 274-3333
**** AD R O W Y B AI CU IV
EA DW TX CI MM OT ****

Janet Zwick, Director
Iowa Department of
  Public Health
Division of Substance Abuse
  and Health Promotion
Lucus State Office Bldg./4th Floor
Des Moines, IA 50319
(515) 281-3641

Kansas
Saint Francis Hospital
Chemical Dependancy
  Treatment Center
1700 West 7th Street
Topeka, Kansas 66606
(913) 295-8360
** AD I O IV TX CI PV OT **

Andrew O'Donavan
Commissioner
Alcohol and Drug Abuse Services
2700 West Sixth Street
Biddle Building
Topeka, Kansas 66606-1861
(913) 296-3925

Facility	State Authority

Kentucky
Charter Hospital of Louiville
Chemical Dependency Unit
1405 Browns Lane
Louisville, KY 40207
(502) 896-0495 Ext. 240
** AD I O IV DT EA TX **

Michael Townsend, Director
Division of Substance Abuse
Dept. for MH - MR Services
275 East Main Street
Frankfort, KY 40621
(502) 564-2880

Louisiana
CPC Meadowood Hospital
Substance Abuse Services
9032 Perkins Road
Baton Rouge, LA 70816
(504) 766-8553
** AD I Y IV DT DW TX CI
PV OT **

Robert A. Perkins, Sr., Secretary
Division of Alcohol and
    Drug Abuse Services
Box 3868
1201 Capital Access Road
Baton Rouge, LA 70821
(504) 342-9350

Maine
Jackson Brook Institute
    Care Unit
175 Running Hill Road
South Portland, ME 04106
(207) 761-2310
** AD I IV DT EA TX **

Neill Miner, Director
Office of Alcoholism and
    Drug Abuse Prevention
Bureau of Rehabilitation
State House Station #11
Augusta, ME 04333
(207) 289-1110

Maryland
Positive Alternative of
Psychological Sevices, Inc.
111 Anapolis Street
Anapolis, MD 21401
(301) 269-6977
** AD O Y IH PI EA DW TX **

Lloyd Sokolow, J.D., Ph.D.
Director Maryland State Drug
    Abuse
    Administration
201 West Preston Street
Baltimore, MD 21202
(301) 225-6925

Massachusetts
Center for Addictive
    Behaviors, Inc.
Detoxification Unit
450 Maple Street
Danvers, MA 01923
(508) 777-2121
** AD R PI IV DT TX OT **

Dave Mulligan, Director
Division of Substance Abuse
    Services
150 Tremont Street
Boston, MA 02111
(617) 727-8614

Facility	State Authority

Michigan
Metro Medical Group East
Chemical Dependency Program
4401 Conner Street
Detroit, MI 48215
(313) 823-9800
** AD O W Y E IV TX **

Ken Eaton, Administrator
Office of Substance
  Abuse Services
Department of Public Health
3423 North Logan Street
Lansing, MI 48909
(517) 335-8809

Minnesota
Riverside Medical Center
Adult Chemical Dependency
  Services
2512 South 7th Street
Minneapolis, MN 55454
(612) 337-4403
** AD I O W Y E IH IV DT EA
TX CI **

Cynthia Turnure, Ph.D., Director
Chemical Dependency
  Program Division
Department of Human Services
444 Lafayette Road
St. Paul, MN 55155-3823
(612) 296-4610

Mississippi
Jackson Recovery Center
5354 I-55 South Frontage Road
Jackson, MS 39212
(601) 372-9788
** AD I R IV DT TX **

Anne D. Robertson, Director
Division of Alcohol and
  Drug Abuse
Department of Mental Health
Robert E. Lee State Office
  Building, 11th Floor
Jackson, MS 39201
(601) 359-1288

Missouri
NASCO Central Clinic
2305 Saint Louis Avenue
Saint Louis, MO 63117
(314) 241-4310
** AD R O W B IV DT DW TX **

Lois Oslon, Director
Division of Alcohol and
  Drug Abuse
Department of Mental Health
1915 South Ridge Drive/Box 687
Jefferson City, MO 65102
(314) 751-4942

Facility	State Authority

Montana
Flathead Valley
Chemical Dependency Clinics, Inc.
38 East Washington Street
Kalispell, MT 59901
(406) 756-6453
** AD O IV EA DW TX PV **

Robert Anderson, Administrator
Alcohol and Drug Abuse Division
   State of Montana
Department of Institutions/Box
   94728
Helena, MT 59601
(406) 444-2827

Nebraska
Lincoln General Hospital
Youth Treatment Services
1630 Lake Street
Lincoln, NE 68502
(402) 473-5394
** AD I O Y IV DT DW TX PV **

Cecilia D. Willis, Ph.D.,
   Director
Division of Alcoholism and
   Drug Abuse
Dept. of Public Institutions, Box
   94728
Lincoln, NE 68509
(402) 471-2851, Ext.: 5583

Nevada
Western Counseling Associates
Adult Residential Program
930 N. 4th Street
Las Vegas, NV 89101
(702) 383-4044
** AD R IV TX **

Richard Ham, Chief Bureau of
   Alcohol and
   Drug Abuse
Department of Human Resources
505 East King Street
Carson City, NV 89710
(702) 885-4790

New Hampshire
Concord Hospital
Alcohol and Drug Abuse Services
250 Pleasant Street
Concord, NH 03301
(603) 225-2711, Ext.: 3101
** AD I IV DT TX CI **

Geraldine Sylvester, Director
Office of Alcohol and Drug
   Abuse Prevention
Health and Welfare Building
Hazen Drive
Concord, NH 03301
(603) 271-6100

Facility	State Authority

New Jersey
Community Guidance Center of
  Mercer County
Substance Abuse Recovery
  Program
2300 Hamilton Avenue
Trenton, NJ 08619
(609) 587-7044
** D O IV EA DW TX PV **

Riley Regan, Director
New Jersey Division of Alcoholism
  and Drug Abuse
129 East Hanover Street
Trenton, NJ 08625
(609) 292-8947

New Mexico
Hogares, Inc.
1218 Griegos Road, NW
Albuquerque, NM 87107
(505) 345-8471
** AD R O Y IV TX **

Kent McGregor, Chief
Substance Abuse Bureau
Behavioral Health
  Services Division
Sante Fe, NM 87504-0968
(505) 827-2601

New York
Community Narcotics
  Prevention Program
119 East 106th Street
New York, NY 10029
(212) 534-2250
** AD W Y E B H CU PV **

Marguerite T. Sanders, Director
New York Division of
  Alcoholism and Alcohol Abuse
194 Washington Avenue
Albany, NY 12210
(518) 474-5417

North Carolina
Charter Northridge Hospital
400 Newton Road
Raleigh, NC 27615
(919) 847-0008
** AD I O IV DT EA DW
TX PV **

William Carroll, Acting Director
Alcohol and Drug Abuse Section
Division of Mental Health &
  Mental Retardation Services
325 North Salisbury Street
Raleigh, NC 27611
(919) 733-4670

Facility	State Authority

North Dakota
Lake Region Human Service
  Center
Alcohol and Drug Unit
Highway 2 West
Devils Lake, ND 58301
(701) 662-7581
** AD O IV EA DW TX CI
PV OT **

John Allen, Director
Division of Alcoholism and
  Drug Abuse
North Dakota Department of
  Human Services
State Capital / Judicial Wing
Bismarck, ND 58505
(701) 224-2769

Ohio
Community Guidance, Inc.
Genesis / A New Beginning
3134 Euclid Avenue
Cleveland, OH 44115 3006
(216) 431-7774
** AD R O W B H AI IH CU IV
TX CI PV **

Suzanne C. Tolbert, Chief
Bureau on Alcohol and Recovery
Ohio Department of Health
170 N. High Street, 3rd Floor
Columbus, OH
(614) 466-3445

Oklahoma
Drug Recovery, Inc.
Counseling Center
6161 North May Avenue
Suite 28
Oklahoma City, OK 73112
(405) 232-9804
** AD O IV EA TX **

Tom Stanitis, Director
Alcohol and Drug Programs
Oklahoma Department of
  Mental Health
P.O. Box 53277, Capital Station
Oklahoma City, OK 73152
(405) 271-7474

Oregon
Buckley House
605 West 4th Street
Eugene, OR 97402
(503) 343-6512
** A OT **

Jeffrey Kushner, Assist. Director
Office of Alcohol and Drug
  Abuse Programs
301 Public Service Building
Salem, OR 97310
(503) 378-2163

Facility	State Authority

Pennsylvania
Saint Joseph Hospital
Detox Unit
250 College Avenue
Lancaster, PA 17604
(717) 291-8449
** AD I IV DT EA TX **

Jeannine Peterson
Deputy Secretary
Drug and Alcohol Programs
Pennsylvania Department
 of Health
Box 90
Harrisburg, PA 17108
(717) 787-9857

Puerto Rico
Modulo De Tratamiento Carcel
Distrito De Ponce
Calle Castillo 34 Esq, Lolita Tizol
Ponce, PR 00731
(809) 844-8155
** D R H IV TX **

Isabel Suliveres de Martinez
Secretary
Department of Anti-Addiction
 Services
Box B-Y, Rio Piedras Station
Rio Piedras, PR 00928
(809) 764-3795

Rhode Island
Community Counseling
 Center, Inc.
Alcohol Treatment Program
160 Beechwood Avenue
Pawtucket, RI 02860
(401) 722-5573
** A O W Y E EA TX CI PV **

William Pimentel, Director
Rhode Island Division of
 Substance Abuse
Administration Building
Cranston, RI 02920
(401) 464-2091

South Carolina
Baker Hospital
Chaps Baker Treatment Center
2750 Speissegger Drive
Charleston, SC 29405
(803) 744-2110
** AD I W Y E IH CU IV DT TX **

William J. McCord, Director
South Carolina Commission on
 Alcohol and Drug Abuse
3700 Forest Drive
Columbia, SC 29204
(803) 734-9520

Facility	State Authority

South Dakota
Carroll Institute
Sioux Falls Detox. Ctr./
   Arch Halfway House
333 South Spring Street
Sioux Falls, SD 57104
(605) 332-9257
** AD R Y E DT TX **

Robert Anderson, Director
Division of Alcohol and
   Drug Abuse
Joe Foss Building
523 East Capital
Pierre, SD 57501
(605) 773-3123

Tennessee
Agape, Inc.
Halfway House
205-211 Scott Avenue, NE
Knoxville, TN 37917
(615) 525-1661
** AD R W IV TX PV **

Rudy Brooms, M.D.
Assistant Commissioner
Alcohol and Drug Abuse
   Services
TN Department of Mental
   Retardation
706 Church Street, 4th Floor
Nashville, TN 37219
(615) 741-1921

Texas
Charlton Methodist Hospital
Alcoholism Dependency
Treatment Center
3500 Wheatland Road
Dallas, Tx 75237
(214) 709-9800
** AD I O IH IV DT TX PV **

Bob Dickson, Executive Director
Texas Commission on Alcohol
   and Drug Abuse
1705 Guadalupe Street
Austin, TX 78701
(512) 463-5510

Trust Territories
Facility not listed,
call your State Authority.

Masao Kumangai, M.D.
Director
Health Services
Offices of the High Commissioner
Saipan, Trust Territories 96950
(615) 741-1921

Facility	State Authority

Utah
Highland Ridge Hospital
Substance Abuse Services
4578 Highland Drive
Salt Lake City, UT 84117
(801) 272-9851
** AD I O W IV DT EA TX CI OT **

Leon PoVey, Director
Division of Substance Abuse
120 N. 200 West, 4th Floor
Box 45500
Salt Lake City, UT 84145-0500
(801) 538-3939

Vermont
Community House
213 Elliot Terrace
Brattleboro, VT 05301
(802) 257-7470
** AD R TX PV **

Richard Powell II, Director
Office of Alcohol and
   Drug Abuse Programs
103 South Maine Street
Waterbury, VT 05676
(802) 241-2170 or 241-1000

Virginia
Arlington Hospital
Addiction Treatment Program
1701 N. George Mason Drive
Arlington, VA 22205
(703) 558-6536
** AD I IV DT TX OT **

Wayne Thacker, Director
Office of Substance
   Abuse Services
State Department of Mental
   Health and Retardation
109 Govenor St./Box 1797
Richmond, VA 23214
(804) 786-3906

Virgin Islands
Facility not listed,
call your State
Authority.

Corrine A. Allen, Ph.D.
Director
Division of Mental Health
   Alcoholism and Dependency
P.O. Box 520
St. Croix, VI 00820
(809) 773-1992

Facility	State Authority

Washington
Ballard Community
  Hospital Careunit
NW Market and Barnes Avenues
Seattle, WA 98107
(206) 789-7209
** AD I IV DT TX CI MM OT **

Ken Stark, Director
Bureau of Alcoholism and
  Substance Abuse
Washington Dept. of Social
  and Health Services
Mail Stop OB-44W
Olympia, WA 98504
(206) 753-5866

West Virginia
Appalachian Regional
  Comprehensive Alcoholism Pro-
  gram
306 Stanaford Road
Beckley, WV 25801
(304) 255-3000, Ext.: 409
** AD I IV DT EA TX OT **

Jack Clohan, Jr., Director
Division of Alcohol and
  Drug Abuse
State Capital
1800 Washington St., East
Room 451
Charleston, WV 25305
(304) 348-2276

Wisconsin
Milwaukee Council on Drug Abuse
1442 North Farwell Avenue
Milwaukee, WI 53202
(414) 271-7822
** AD Y H PV OT **

Larry Monson, ACSW
Director
Office of Alcohol and Other
  Drug Abuse
1 West Wilson Street
Box 7851
Madison, WI 53707
(608) 266-3442

Wyoming
De Paul Hospital
Chemical Dependency Center
2600 East 18th Street
Cheyenne, WY 82001
(307) 632-6411, Ext. 664
** AD I IV DT EA DW TX **

Jean Defratis, Director
Alcohol and Drug Abuse
  Programs
Hathaway Building
Cheyenne, WY 82002
(307) 777-6494

Source: National Directory of Drug Abuse and Alcoholism Treatment and Prevention Programs, 1989. (Data updated for accuracy). U.S. Department of Health and Human Services, Public Health Service. Alcohol, Drug Abuse, and Mental Health Administration. National Institute on Drug Abuse. National Institute on Alcohol Abuse and Alcoholism.

Updated for accuracy.

15/What Can I Do To Help?

Some Suggestions

- After learning the facts about AIDS, use what you know to protect yourself.

- Share this information with your children and other family members, friends, and co-workers.

- Do not share needles or engage in risky sexual behaviors.

- Teach your children compassion. Your child may know someone who has AIDS.

- Show support and understanding for people who are infected with the HIV and for those who have AIDS. Keep in mind that you can not get HIV/AIDS from being a friend.

- Encourage teachers and administrators to provide AIDS education in your child's school.

- Become a volunteer. Get involved with your local Red Cross or AIDS service organization to learn more about what you can do to help raise community awareness, prevent the spread of HIV infection or provide care for those infected or ill.

- Donate blood or help sponsor a blood drive.

- Make sure you meet donor requirements before donating blood. Then, let others know that it is impossible for a donor to get infected with HIV/AIDS by donating blood. When healthy donors give blood, it saves lives.

- Donate money or sponsor an AIDS fund raising event.

Summary

Obviously, AIDS (Acquired Immune Deficiency Syndrome) is a disease which all of us should know about. It is not a disease which is exclusive to any one group of people. It will take years of research in order to come up with a cure, and education will sustain the uninfected portion of our population in the interim period.

Sexual and drug practices have to be altered, and in some cases discontinued, in order to prevent the spread of infection.

Adults, after learning the facts, need to spread this information around to families (including children), to friends and associates. Intravenous drug abusers at every level have to be informed of the facts about AIDS.

The good news concerning AIDS is that you don't have to get it. It is something that can be avoided if you know and put to use the facts.

Bibliography

Books:
AIDS, edited by Robert Emmet Long, The Reference Shelf, The H.W. Wilson Company, 1987.

AIDS, The Mystery & the Solution, The New Epidemic of Acquired Immune Deficiency Syndrome, by Alan Cantwell, Jr., M.D., Second Edition, Revised, Aries Rising Press, 1986.

AIDS, The Ultimate Challenge, by Elisabeth Kubler-Ross, M.D., Macmillan Publishing Company, 1987.

AIDS: Trading Fears for Facts, A Guide for Teens, by Karen Hein, M.D., Theresa Foy Digeronimo and the Editors of Consumer Reports Books, Consumers Union of the United States, Inc., 1989.

Crisis, Heterosexual Behavior in The Age of AIDS, by William H. Masters, M.D., Virginia E. Johnson, and Robert C. Kolodny, M.D., Grove Press, Inc., 1988.

"Does AIDS Hurt?", Educating Young Children About AIDS, Suggestions for Teachers, Parents and Other Care Providers of Children to Age 10, by Marcia Quackenbush, MS and Sylvia Villarreal, MD, Network Publications, a division of ETR Associates, 1988.

The Essential AIDS Fact Book, What You Need to Know to Protect Yourself, Your Family, All Your Loved Ones, prepared in cooperation with the Columbia University Health Service by Paul Harding Douglas and Laura Pinsky, Pocket Books, a division of Simon and Schuster, Inc., 1987.

Mobilizing Against AIDS, Revised and Enlarged Edition, prepared in cooperation with The Institute of Medicine, National Academy of Sciences, by Eve K. Nichols, Harvard University Press, 1989.

Questions & Answers on AIDS, by Lyn Robert Frumkin, M.D., Ph.D. and John Martin Leonard, M.D., Avon Publishers, 1987.

The Real Truth About Women and AIDS: How to Eliminate the Risks Without Giving Up Love and Sex, by Helen Singer Kaplan, M.D., Ph.D., Simon and Schuster, Inc., 1987.

Safe Sex in a Dangerous World, Understanding and Coping with the Threat of AIDS, by Art Ulene, M.D., Vintage Books, 1987.

Safe Sex in the Age of AIDS, For Men and Women, prepared by the Institute for the Advanced Study of Human Sexuality, Citadel Press, 1986.

Teen Guide to Safe Sex, by Alan E. Nourse, M.D., published in U.S. by Franklin Watts, 1988.

The Truth About AIDS, Evolution of An Epidemic, revised and updated, by Ann Giudici Fettner and William A. Check, Ph.D., Henry Holt and Company, 1985.

You Can Do Something About AIDS, edited by Sasha Alyson, A public service project of the publishing industry, The Stop AIDS project, Inc., 1988.

What We Need to Know About AIDS Now! The AIDS File, by George Jacobs and Joseph Kerrins, M.D., Cromlech Books, Inc., 1987.

Centers for Disease Control (CDC) Publications:

CDC, MMWR (Morbidity and Mortality Weekly Report), AIDS and Human Immunodeficiency Virus Infection in the United States: 1988 Update: U.S. Department of Health and Human Services, Vol. 38 / No. S-4, May 12 1989.

CDC, MMWR (Morbidity and Mortality Weekly Report), Human Immunodeficiency Virus Infection in the United States: A Review of Current Knowledge: U.S. Department of Health and Human Services, Vol. 36 / No. S-6, December 18, 1987.

The American National Red Cross (ANRC) Publications:

May 1989: ANRC, HIV Infection and AIDS, Stock No. 329560.
July 1989: ANRC, Emergency and Public Safety Workers and HIV/AIDS-A Duty to Respond, Stock No. 329544.
November 1988: ANRC, Men, Sex, and AIDS, Stock No. 329535.
ANRC, Women, Sex, and AIDS, Stock No. 329537.
ANRC, Children, Parents and AIDS, Stock No. 329540.
ANRC, AIDS and Children, Stock No. 329505.
ANRC, Teenagers and AIDS, Stock No. 329536.
ANRC, Drugs, Sex and AIDS, Stock No. 329539.
ANRC, School Systems and AIDS, Information For Teachers and School Officials, Stock No. 329541.
ANRC, Your Job and AIDS: Are There Risks?, Stock No. 329502.
January 1987: ANRC and U.S Public Health Service, AIDS and Safety of the Nation's Blood Supply, Stock No. AIDS-13.
AIDS: Know the Facts and Resources in Our Community, 1987

San Francisco AIDS Foundation (SFAF) Publications:

SFAF, AIDS Lifeline, The Best Defense Against AIDS Is Information: Copyright 1987, Second Edition, 1989.

SFAF, AIDS Kills Women and Babies, 1988.

SFAF, AIDS in the Workplace, A Guide for Employees: Published 1986, Revised August 1987.

SFAF, Women and AIDS, 3rd Edition, Generic Version, 1987.

SFAF, Sharing Needles Can Give You AIDS, 1987.

SFAF, AIDS Antibody Testing At Alternative Test Sites: Published June, 1985, Revised, 1987.

SFAF, Pregnancy and AIDS, Generic Version, 1st Edition, February 1988.

SFAF, Your Child and AIDS, A Simple Guide For Parents With Children in Daycare and Public Schools. Generic Version, 3rd edition, 1989, 1988.

SFAF, Talking With Your Teen About AIDS, AIDS Lifeline, 1988.

SFAF, IMPETUS, Teaching Parents about "Talking with Teens" and Teaching Teens About Risky Business, October 1988.

SFAF, Alcohol, Drugs and AIDS, 1988.

SFAF, BETA (Bulletin of Experimental Treatments for AIDS): November 1988.

SFAF, Safe sex For Gay and Bisexual Men, Man to Man: 1st Edition, October 1988.

SFAF, An Important Message for Gay & Bisexual Men.

SFAF, Condoms For Couples, 1st Edition, February 1988.

SFAF, Fact vs. Fiction, Ten Things You Should Know About AIDS.

Other Publications:

Sacramento AIDS Foundation, Poppers, Your Health... and AIDS...Can you Afford the Risk?, 1985.

Surgeon General's Report on Acquired Immune Deficiency Syndrome, U.S. Department of Health and Human Services, 1986.

Network Publications: a division of ETR Associates, Santa Cruz, CA, Teens & AIDS, why risk it, Title #161, 1987.

New Body Magazine Special Publication: AIDS Update, New Body Publishing Corp., New York, NY, No. 1 02422, Vol. 2, No. 1, 1988.

Glossary

A

AIDS—Acquired Immune Deficiency Syndrome: a viral disease that attacks the human body's immune system.

AIDS Virus—Human Immunodeficiency Virus (HIV): the virus that is passed through the body fluids of HIV-infected people, and eventually destroys the cells that defend the body.

Antibodies: a protein made by the immune system to destroy invaders and fight infection.

Antigens: a foreign substance that stimulates the immune system.

Analingus: oral-anal sex; also called "rimming."

ARC—AIDS-Related Complex: a condition caused by the AIDS virus (HIV) in which the patient tests positive for AIDS infection and has a specific set of clinical symptoms.

Artificial insemination: introduction of semen into the uterus or oviduct by other than natural means.

Autoimmune diseases: those diseases caused by the immune system attacking its own tissues.

Autologus: a blood transfusion in which a person's own blood is drawn in advance and stored for upcoming surgery.

AZT—Azidothymedine: a drug used in the treatment of AIDS patients. It stops the multiplication of the AIDS virus inside the cell.

B

B-cells: cells that function as the "antibody" or "humoral" system. They are instructed to produce antibodies by the branch of the T-family known as T-helpers.

Biopsy: removal of a tissue sample in order to diagnose a disease.

Bisexual: relating to, or exhibiting sexual desire toward members of both sexes.

C

Cancer: a group of diseases in which abnormal cells grow uncontrollably.

These cells can destroy surrounding tissue and spread to other parts of the body.

Casual Contact: non-sexual contact or association; everyday contact, such as a hug, a handshake or using a drinking fountain.

Cesarean birth: surgical incision of the walls of the abdomen and uterus for delivery of offspring.

Condom: a sheath commonly made of latex material, which is worn over the penis. (used to prevent AIDS and other sexually transmitted diseases, as well as conception)

Congenital: existing or dating from birth; such as congenital AIDS.

Contagious: can be spread indirectly or directly. A contagious disease can be passed from one person to another through the air as well as by touch. AIDS is not contagious in this sense, because it requires an actual exchange of body fluid.

Cunnilingus: oral-vaginal sex.

D

Dementia: a loss of mental capacity. AIDS-related dementia may be caused by the HIV or other infections.

Directed donation: the option of having someone you know donate blood for you, which would be used for elective surgery.

Dormant: a state of suspended activity.

DNA: material in the nucleus of a cell which contains the cell's genetic code.

E

ELIZA—Enzyme-Linked Immunosorbent Assay: the basic blood test used to detect the particular antibodies that react to the HIV. If the result of the ELIZA test is negative, it indicates that there are no HIV antibodies present at the time of the test. If positive, further testing must be done to establish the presence of the AIDS virus.

Epidemic: a disease which effects many people at one time.

Epidemiology: the study of disease patterns. Especially important in tracking AIDS is the relationship between age, location and sexual habits of people.

Etiology: the cause and origin of disease.

F

Fellatio: oral-penile sex.

Fisting: insertion of the fingers or entire hand into the anus.

G

Germicide: an agent that destroys germs.

Gonorrhea: an infectious disease of the rectum and cervix caused by a bacterium and transmitted chiefly by sexual intercourse.

H

Hemophilia: a hereditary blood-clotting disfunction that requires the administration of a clotting factor derived from the blood of donors. It can cause serious internal bleeding. Hemophiliacs are also known as "bleeders" and are almost exclusively male. They bruise easily and bleed profusely.

Hepatitis: inflammation of the liver, resulting in jaundice, loss of appetite, malaise, fever and abdominal pain.

Heterosexual: relating to, or exhibiting sexual desire toward a member of the opposite sex.

HIV-Human Immunodeficiency Virus: see AIDS virus.

HIV Encephalopathy: a disease in which the HIV invades the brain, causing dementia.

HIV Wasting Disease: AIDS-related disease, characterized by weight loss.

Homosexual; relating to, or exhibiting sexual desire toward a member of one's own sex.

I

Immune system: the body's defense mechanism for resisting disease.

IRA—Immunofluorescence and Radioimmunoprecipitation Assays: tests used to deny or confirm the presence of the AIDS virus in a person's blood when a combination of ELISA and the Western blot proves indeterminate.

Incubation Period: the period between exposure to an infection and the development of symptoms of the disease (in the case of AIDS, five to ten years).

IV Drug User, intravenous drug user: a person who injects drugs into his/her bloodstream, using hypodermic needles and syringes. Illegal IV drug use is thought to be the main avenue of the AIDS virus to the heterosexual population.

K

KS—Kaposi's Sarcoma: a tumor of the walls of blood vessels. It usually appears as pink to purple, painless spots on the surface of the skin, but can also occur internally. KS is one of the major infections found among PWA (people with AIDS), especially gay and bisexual men.

L

Lymph nodes: glands that fight infection by filtering microorganisms and producing antibodies to fight them. These glands become swollen when disease conditions exist in the body.

M

Masturbation: the manipulation of the genitals for sexual gratification.

Monogamy: the state of being married to one person at a time. Less specifically, in the context of AIDS, it refers to sustaining an intimate relationship with one person at a time.

O

Opportunistic Diseases: fatal and otherwise rare diseases that are contracted, in this case, by AIDS victims, and that eventually kill the victim (rare cancers, infections, etc.).

Oral Intercourse: see: cunnilingus, fellatio, and analingus.

P

Poppers: the slang term for a mixture of chemicals used as an inhalant to achieve a "high" during sex and often during social events such as dancing. The active ingredients are amyl and butyl nitrate, which damage the body's ability to stay healthy.

Pepi-T: a drug developed for the treatment of AIDS patients. It blocks the virus' entry into the cell, binds to the cell surface and blocks access of the virus to white cell replication.

Prophylactic: a drug or device that helps to prevent a disease before it occurs.

PCP: drug often used by IV drug abusers.

PWA: Person With AIDS or Persons With AIDS.

R

Retrovirus: a special kind of RNA virus which works in backward fashion. It converts genetic information into DNA. (Usually genetic information goes from DNA to RNA, therefore, the "retro" prefix.)

S

Slipping: slang term, meaning occasional unsafe sex.

Spermicide: a sperm-killing medication used to prevent pregnancy. Spermicides take one of four forms: foam, jelly, cream, and suppositories. Nonoxynol-9 is the most widely used sperm killing agent in the United States. Benzalkonium chloride, reputedly a more powerful spermicide, is available in France, Canada, Spain, Switzerland and parts of Africa, but not in the U.S. Both kill the AIDS virus.

Safe Sex: sex which is performed using measures and controls to prevent the spread of AIDS and other STDs.

Signs and Symptoms: medically speaking, signs are the manifestation of the illness you have and symptoms are what you tell the doctor you are suffering from.

STD: sexually transmitted disease, a disease usually transmitted through sexual behavior.

Syndrome: an illness that has distinct signs and symptoms but does not have a known cause.

Syphilis: an ancient and deadly sexually transmitted disease caused by a germ called spirochete.

T

T-Cells: a group of lymphocytes (white blood cells) that help control how fast or slow the B-cells make antibodies to fight and infection. T-cells are the specific cells killed by the AIDS virus.

Thymus: a gland in the neck that is essential to the production of T-cells.

Transfusion: the introduction of solution into a person's blood stream. Some prople have become infected with the AIDS virus through transfusion of HIV-infected blood.

Transmit: to cause or allow to spread from one person to another.

U

Unsafe sex: unprotected sex with no regard for the presence of HIV/AIDS and other STDs.

V

Vaccine: a matter or preparation which is administered to produce or artificially increase immunity to a particular disease.

Venereal: a word meaning "sexually related" and derived from Venus, the goddess of love.

Viral disease: illness caused by a virus. Unlike bacterial diseases, which can be cured, viral diseases can be reduced in severity by our immune systems, but not removed from our bodies once "exposed." AIDS is a viral disease.

Virus: the smallest of the microorganisms that cause infections in humans. These are technically parasites, because they depend on living host cells for survival. Viruses cause many illnesses, including the common cold, measles, mumps and chicken pox.

W

Water Sports: slang term for sexual behavior characterized by urinating on partner.

Western Blot: a test used to back up an ELIZA blood test when it gives a positive result; that is, when it indicates the presence of the AIDS virus in the blood.

White cells: blood components essential to our immune system, and prime targets of the AIDS virus.

Works: slang term for drug paraphernalia (needles, syringes, cotton, etc.).

Index

Page references in *italics* refer to figures and tables.

K

Karposi's Sarcoma, 2, 84

L

Latex condoms, 13-16, 82
Living with AIDS
    interviews, 45-54
Long-time association, 17
Lubricants, 14

M

Men and AIDS, 29-31
    Male adult/adolescent AIDS
        cases, *31*
Minority Task Force on AIDS, 59
Monogamy, 12, 84

N

National AIDS Information
Hotline—
    U.S. Public Health Service, 58
Nation's blood supply, 24-25
National Coalition of Gay
    Sexually Transmitted Disease
    Services, 59
National Drug Treatment Referral
    Hotline, 60
Nonoxynol-9, 13
Needles, 3, 6, 12, 13
    disposable, 12, 19
    how to clean, *18*
    how to dispose of, 19
    packaged and sanitized, 19
    tattoo, 12

O

Opportunistic, 1, 84
Oral sex, 4, 84
Opportunistic diseases, 84
    Karposi's Sarcoma, 2, 84
    Pneumocystis Carinii Pneu-
        monia, 2
Other STDs and AIDS, 44
Oral intercourse, 4, 84

P

Partner's faithfulness, 11
Pediatric AIDS cases, *37*
Percentages of AIDS cases
    by category, 5
Percentages of IV-drug users
    cleaning equipment, *19*
Poppers, 26, 27
Prevention, 11-19
    discussing AIDS with sexual
        partner, 11
    right to ask questions, 11
Projected numbers AIDS cases:
    1989-1993, *3*

R

Results of HIV-antibody testing, 8, 9
Rights
    to ask questions of partner, 11
    to anonymity in testing, 9

S

Safe behavior, 12
San Francisco AIDS Foundation, 59

About the Author

Brenda Smith Faison is the president and founder of Designbase Publishing (a division of Designbase Associates, Incorporated) in Durham, North Carolina.

From 1982 to 1985 she worked for IBM in corporate publications, design and graphics. In 1985 she formed Designbase Associates, an advertising and graphic design firm. She taught for three years at her alma mater and has lectured at North Carolina State University.

She received her Bachelor of Arts degree from North Carolina Central University at Durham, with a concentration in visual communications. She obtained her Master of Product Design degree, with a concentration in visual design, from North Carolina State's prestigious School of Design at Raleigh. Ms. Faison is married, and is the mother of five-year-old twin girls.

Prior to her work on The AIDS Handbook, Ms. Faison published an innovative series of posters which speak to the drug and alcohol abuse dilemma now facing our country. This series is currently in use nationally in schools, universities, corporations, treatment clinics, military bases and government agencies.

Ms. Faison's approach to The AIDS Handbook is that of a layperson in consultation with medical and education professionals, and related organizations and agencies. Her point of view synthesizes essential information, allowing the facts presented here to be of service to people at every level. She strongly believes that everyone, of all professions and backgrounds, has something to contribute to the fight against AIDS.

About the Editor

Dr. Laila Moustafa is president of Human and Environmental Health International. She received her bachelor's degree in engineering from the renowned Cairo University, at Cairo, Egypt. Her Master's in education and sciences, she obtained from California Polytechnic State University, at San Luis Obispo. Dr. Moustafa further studied at Washington State University, at Pullman, where she received her Doctorate of Sciences degree. Dr. Moustafa has also obtained her PDF in developmental biology from the University of Pennsylvania, at Philadelphia.

She is the recipient of several awards including the UAR Fellowship, the NIH-Postdoctoral Fellowship, and the Alexander von Humboldt-Stiftung Fellowship.

Shortly after the receipt of her doctorate, she worked with the National Institute of Environmental Health Sciences for five years in the United States, and four years in Germany. During this time she developed several pioneer research programs in the field of biotechnology, cloning, sex determination, embryo transfer and twining; and has authored and co-authored some 50 scientific papers on these subjects. She has lectured at several universities in various countries, including the United States, Germany, Austria, Italy, and Egypt.

Dr. Moustafa joined the United Nation's World Health Organization in 1980, where she was instrumental in establishing the Interregional Research Unit in the U.S. This was an extension the International Program on Chemical Safety Central Unit in Geneva. In 1987, she accepted the leadership role in her current post (president of Human and Environmental Health International), an organization through which her work has spanned six continents.

Dr. Moustafa is an advocate of a systematic approach to bringing concerned individuals and agencies together with current vital knowledge and the status of events. She has been working with several Red Cross chapters in the Eastern North Carolina Territory; initiating HIV/AIDS education programs that meet the community's needs. As an educator she trains facilitators and instructors to reach out to all community members. Her involvement is an ongoing process.